LONG JOURNEY

CONTEMPORARY

NORTHWEST POETS

EDITED *by* DAVID BIESPIEL

Oregon State University Press
Corvallis, Oregon

The paper in this book meets the guidelines for permanence and durability of the Committee on Production Guidelines for Book Longevity of the Council on Library Resources and the minimum requirements of the American National Standard for Permanence of Paper for Printed Library Materials Z39.48-1984.

Library of Congress Cataloging-in-Publication Data

Long Journey: Contemporary Northwest poets / edited by David Biespiel.
     p. cm.
    An anthology of contemporary American and Canadian poets from Alaska, Oregon, Washington, Montana, Idaho, and British Columbia.
    ISBN-13: 978-0-87071-098-8 (alk. paper)
    ISBN-10: 0-87071-098-2 (alk. paper)
    1. American poetry—Northwestern States. 2. Canadian poetry--British Columbia. 3. Northwestern States--Poetry. 4. British Columbia—Poetry. 5. American poetry—20th century. 6. American poetry—21st century. 7. Canadian poetry—20th century. 8. Canadian poetry—21st century. I. Biespiel, David, 1964–
    PS570.C62 2006
    811'.60809795—dc22

                                    2006010278

Cover and text design by Jennifer Viviano

OREGON STATE UNIVERSITY PRESS
500 Kerr Administration
Corvallis OR 97331-2122
541-737-3166 • fax 541-737-3170
http://oregonstate.edu/dept/press

FOR MY MOTHER AND FATHER

In the long journey out of the self,
There are many detours, washed-out interrupted raw places
Where the shale slides dangerously
And the back wheels hang almost over the edge
At the sudden veering, the moment of turning.
Better to hug close, wary of rubble and falling stones.

—*Theodore Roethke, "North American Sequence"*

⊞ CONTENTS

❈ FOREWORD

There is no such thing as regional poetry. If there were—and if there were some Politburic consensus on what that school of poetry might include (grits, freeways, and Robert E. Lee, say, for the Southern School or rain, trees, and salmon for the Northwest School)—then no self-respecting poet would want to write it anyway.

Certainly a good critic has a need, even obligation to classify Isms, Schools, and Styles. But poets don't work that way. A poet doesn't sit down at the writing desk in the wee hours of the morning, with the sun barely blinking, and the coffee not yet brewed, and the house just beginning to warm, and think, Well, today, by God, I'm going to write another Southeastern Alaska poem. At least, I hope not.

The poet who remains in a single region from cradle to grave, or even in a single village as Emily Dickinson did in Amherst, Massachusetts, might be more inclined to write out of a regional predicament than the poet who has uprooted and moved around. On the other hand, the poet who has lived in one region throughout his or her life might easily reject that region's literary manners, habits, and clichés (again, think Emily Dickinson). Then, there's the poet who long ago left a region and—as the decades go by—still writes about that former place with integrity and urgency.

Today's immense dissemination of the written word and decent availability of books in translation—not to mention the peculiarities of a single poet's imagination—make a purely provincial aesthetic nearly impossible to achieve. This is a continent where mobility is the demographic norm and enormous quantities of information, knowledge, and experience are easily accessible and transferable, so to say that a poet's entire sense of poetic language or temperament is completely tethered to a single geographical place is to observe something so unlikely as to render the point irrelevant. Given the mixture of this region's urban dynamism, suburban heartiness and sprawl, and rural calm, could one ever make a claim for a single Northwest aesthetic—or as I have heard some suggest, that there is a particular Northwest U.S. aesthetic as opposed to a particular Northwest Canadian aesthetic? Certainly anyone should feel free to proclaim that Poet X or Poet Y is...well, a Northwest Poet. But no poet would want to be labeled with such pseudo-aesthetic finality. Can you blame them? A poet's interests in the sublime, in the ambiguity and contours of language, in all the themes available for a poet to explore, naturally lie far beyond place alone.

What I'm questioning here is what is commonly called Poetry of Place. "Society depends on the poet to witness something," Robert Pinsky once said, "and yet the poet can discover that thing only by looking away from what society has learned to see poetically." The same holds for a region. A poet living in the Northwest, for example, discovers and becomes the thing that makes him or her a Northwest poet by looking away from the received preconceptions of what regional writing means. In so doing, a poet learns to see not with a regional sensibility but with a poetic one.

Put another way, consider one of the region's celebrated poets, William Stafford. William Stafford is one of the finest Oregon poets that the state of Kansas ever produced. To read Stafford closely is to be confronted with a wild—though sometimes suburban—Northwestern landscape from a poet who has a Midwesterner's predisposition. That disposition was formed in the progressive populism of a Kansas prairie upbringing. In the late seventies Stafford wrote that when we write we "venture into an immediate engagement with the language we happen to have." Same is true for the region a poet happens to have. William Stafford didn't use poetry to explore the region of the Northwest. The Northwest is just one of the things he used in order to write poetry.

So, do we define regional poetry by what is seen by a poet or how it's seen? And does it really matter if we answer that question? Probably not. To most readers, I'm sure, what matters are the poems. It's for this reason, among others, that the book you're holding is not entitled *Contemporary Northwest Poetry*. No such thing exists. A poet doesn't merely receive the images and subjects a region offers, but transforms them, and in so doing—as in the Heisenberg principle—changes his or her environment. Which is to say that a Northwest poet's impact on our sense of how we see the Northwest may be greater than the Northwest's impact on the poet. "The local is not a place," Robert Creeley once said, "but a place in a given man—what part of it he has been compelled or else brought by love to give witness to in his own mind."

Another example of what I mean might be found in the circumstance of Theodore Roethke, a poet who is a major influence on many of the poets collected here. By the time Theodore Roethke arrived in Seattle in 1947 to teach at the University of Washington, he was 39 years old, had published two highly praised books of poetry, and both his sense of himself as a poet and his compositional habits were more or less fixed. Roethke was born and reared in Saginaw, Michigan, where his father (who died less than a month before Roethke's 15th birthday) operated a greenhouse. At the time he moved West, Roethke was living in State College, Pennsylvania, and before that in Vermont. Given these facts—and that some of his strongest influences are William Blake, Robert Graves, W.B. Yeats, and Dylan Thomas (not an American in the lot), one could not view Theodore Roethke, at mid-career, in the late 1940s and early 1950s, as a Northwest Poet.

In fact, he was only mildly impressed by what he found in post-War Seattle anyway: "The town, its mores (so *damned* genteel—the pioneers are all dead or in jail)—the town, I say, is the worst bore in the U.S.: not a decent restaurant, nothing but beauty parlors and 'smart' shops and toothy dames with zinc curls." By the early sixties he would say that Seattle was simply "ugly."

He hadn't planned to stay in the West. He wanted to move back to the East Coast, to what he felt were the more vibrant centers of literary America. But he did stay. And, without a doubt, the "North-West," as he called it, became a fructifying landscape for his sublime aesthetic—but no more so than the glass-covered ecosystem of the greenhouses of his childhood about which he wrote with distinct and equal interest. In the sixteen years Roethke lived in Seattle, until his death in 1963, he wrote several more books, taught regularly at the University, and influenced so many poets by force of his personality, his exceptional teaching, and his dynamic poetry that if one must use the term

Northwest Poetry, there's a case to be made that Theodore Roethke is the modern father of it.

I'm not suggesting that place didn't matter to Roethke. Certainly it did—"There are those to whom place is unimportant, / But this place, where sea and fresh water meet, / Is important." To one degree or another, place matters to all writers, chiefly as a result of attentiveness and intimacy with the patterns of one's nearest environment. But imagination and invention are crucial, as well. As the British-born poet Denise Levertov once asked (Levertov, by the way, lived in Seattle the last eight years of her life), "Without Attention—to the world outside us, to the voices within us—what poems could possibly come into existence?" Thinking of Roethke, if one were to look closely at his poetry after he moved to Seattle, one would find so many sources beyond the regional ones, so many things to which he gave his "Attention," that it becomes dicey at best to call him, with strict finality, a Northwest Poet.

Feel free to, of course. It makes for good shorthand in discussing poets. I grew up in Houston, and when I first moved to the Pacific Northwest, just by coincidence the promotional materials were being prepared for my first book of poems. The opening sentence of the book's press release proclaimed me a "Northwest nature poet." Though I pointed out to my publisher that I hadn't written even a single poem in the book while living in the Northwest, what he said to me was, "You're there now, so you're one of them." OK, I said, but make it say that I write "Northwest poetry . . . Texas-style."

The danger with outlining a regional aesthetic can be thought of another way, as well. Linda Bierds and Tess Gallagher are poets who have called this region home almost their entire lives. Bierds was born in Wilmington, Delaware and grew up in Anchorage and Seattle. Gallagher is a native. Today they live only 70 miles apart, one on Bainbridge Island, the other in Port Angeles. But their aesthetics as poets, what their poetry looks like, feels like, what the experience is like to read these two poets, is more like 70,000 miles apart. Bierds dwells in realms of the historic and dramatic monologue. Gallagher works in the vineyard of the autobiographical lyric. By any measure, a fair reading of these two poets could no more claim that each writes out of a shared regional experience than to say that the sun comes up in the west.

At the time this anthology was prepared, the Pacific Northwest is where all these poets make their homes and make their art—and this fact is reflected in one of the anthology's rejected titles, *Poets of the Pacific Northwest—for Now*. The goal for compiling this anthology has not been to see how the region defines its poets or even to see if the poets define this region. To curate with a strict regional bias in subject matter would be reductive and would have created a terrible collection of poems. Instead, the anthology is an early 21st century snapshot of how various and engaging this region's poetry is. This anthology, then, is meant as a showcase that exhibits what poets living in this region are working on right now—as a defining moment in the history of the art.

Of the poets in this book, there are those who were born and grew up in the Northwest and have lived here more or less their entire lives. Additionally, there are those who arrived here as children with their parents or, like Theodore Roethke or William Stafford, moved here later in life. They come from places such as Whiting, Indiana; Thomaston, Georgia; Detroit, Michigan, Hanover, New Hampshire; Reading, Pennsylvania; Swift Coast, Saskatchewan; Iowa City, Iowa; and Long Island, New York. Whatever the biographical or historical circumstances of their arrival in the Northwest, however much they have adopted this region or resisted it, all the poets collected here, in the words of Adrienne Rich, confront what all poets confront: "problems of language and style, problems of energy and survival."

Concerned with the whole of living—with the poems being investigations, sometimes transformations of the various elements of living—a poet has many sources and resources. A poet kneads metaphor and imagination as a means to consider, though seldom to completely answer two questions: what does it mean to be human and what is the world? For some the consideration is cause for exaltation. For others, skepticism. But whether they were born in the Pacific Northwest or came to this region later in life, each of the poets in this anthology have one thing in common. Their poems consist of particular and individual records of the long journey of being alive in this age.

Note

Over a hundred poets from Alaska, British Columbia, Idaho, Oregon, Washington, and Western Montana—poets who have published at least one book of poems with a national press—were asked to submit new and if possible unpublished poems for consideration for this anthology. Only a very few poets submitted work from previously published books—typically because they had just published a book and didn't have new poems. Each poet was asked to send up to ten poems, and I made selections based on what came in the door. What I was looking for is what I'm always looking for in poetry: form, honesty, linguistic energy, passion, and the intangible feeling that the poem is coming off the page.

The limitations and failures of this book—including omissions, including taste, including anything at all you might think of that merits hauling me out to the woodshed—are entirely mine. It's worth noting that some poets chose not to participate. In addition, the criteria for being considered for possible inclusion—at least one book of poems with a national press—was arbitrary. But it was necessary, too, because it permits the anthology to be more than simply a personal selection. Naturally, that decision omitted poets. That's not inhumane, but it's regrettable.

A word, too, about the biographical details on the poets: Typically anthologies provide the professional accessories of today's poet, with an emphasis on awards, prizes, medals, and ribbons. Plough through enough of these self-proclamations, and all the accolades—from Third Honorable Mention for the Pond Scum Prize to recipient of the McArthur Fellowship—begin to sound alike, and they are generally uninformative for the general reader or student. The brief biographical sketches offered here might be no better (my intention had been that they run with the poems, but space considerations have forced them to the rear of the book). I hope these sketches seem personal and distinct, and at the very least, more interesting to read than the usual fare. For those wishing to explore more poetry from any of these poets—and an anthology really serves the purpose of directing readers to find more work by the poets whom they enjoy—a broad, though non-scholarly, list of publications for each poet is provided.

—DB

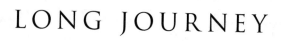

LONG JOURNEY

Jan Lee Ande

CORNERS OF THE MOUTH

Her hands loosen the warm musty smell of soil.
Fingers untangle roots, tug at weeds.

Snap peas twine their tendrils onto lattice
and seeds ride inside green canoes.

Carrots burrow their taproots into earth.
Red chard raises veined hands in the wind.

Thick stalks lift the heavy heads of cauliflower
(those rough orbs white as moons).

She can taste fear in meat, muscle stringy
and bitter, marrow with its history of loss.

Animals visit her dreams, ascend the chute.
Yowls thicken in her throat.

Picking up a sharp stick, she draws two thin
lines of an open mouth gaping

scrapes a space from fibers
scratched out of sand and particles of grit.

A REMEDY, WITHHELD

Here leopard's bane wanders eyebright
near leafblade and grass. Mender of muddled
blood and horrors stored in muscle.

Arnica montana. Narrow leaves reach out
and from their center a stalk
a foot or two high bears a yellow flower.

Jews were forced to wear a yellow star:
its six points stitched onto armbands
and badges, the left side of coats.

Wanting a word of sorrow, mournful
heart, he walked along a path with no one
through the Black Forest to the hut.

There he found a well—yellow star shape
hung above. Signing the visitors book
meant nothing. Silence was drowning.

After leaves die down, gather the roots.
From rootstalk (dark brown and rounded)
fibers spring like wiry threads.

Add spirits to mix a tincture for wounds.
Rub oil onto skin thin as lampshades.
Seal their feet. Anoint all those souls.

Ginger Andrews

WHERE WE MESSED UP

in our thinking, I tell my sister,
was believing that the last thing
we wanted from a man
was to have him worship
the ground we walk on.

There is nothing wrong
with having car doors
opened for you, I say,
there is nothing wrong
with a man who rubs
your back before you rub his,
or, even if you don't.

What's wrong with a man
who cooks, I ask, or a man
who irons your blouse
before he irons his own shirt—
not that anyone irons anymore,
but you get my point. How about
a man who mows the yard,
cleans out the gutters,
checks your oil and airs up your tires—
tires that barely need air . . . Yeah,
I know, I know, my sister says,

I can't believe I never
prayed for a praying man,
one who'd actually get on his knees,
wash my feet sometimes, you know,
sit me down on the sofa, take my shoes off,
call me doll face, peaches, angel eyes.

Judith Barrington

IMAGINARY ISLANDS

St. Brandan's, Atlantis, Macy's and Swain's
are islands that never stayed still on the map:
a shape in the mind is all that remains

though the sailor who saw one would rack his brains
to remember the moment he threw up his cap
and shouted Land Ho! at Macy's or Swain's.

Cartographers drew them beside their new names
as a circle or crescent, a leaf or a cup
but a shape in the mind is all that remains

of that rock that loomed from torrential rains
or parted the clouds then slid back through the gap:
Was it Macy's, St Brandan's, Atlantis or Swain's

or some other echo a body retains
from those months in a warm sea, rocking asleep?
A shape in the mind is all that remains

as we boot our computers and run for our trains
or finger brochures for a long, slow, sea trip
to St. Brandan's, Atlantis, Macy's or Swain's
in search of the shape which is all that remains.

Judith Barrington

SOULS UNDER WATER

No longer tumbled by currents as when
long ago they were lodgers in frail bodies,
now they drift free of the flesh that was sucked
and nibbled from bones and the blood that swirled
away, its quick red streaking the deeps.

Souls mingle in the democracy of weed.
Passing through great barnacled bulkheads
once-passengers, transparent without furs or jewels,
glide through the shiver that marks the presence
of stoker or convict, or the drunken oilman

who one night staggered to the edge of the spider-legged rig
and dreaming of his girlfriend—unusually tender
in his mind at that dizzy moment—plunged through cans
and plastic trash, into the arms of another.
Welcome, said the souls, though his ears heard nothing.

No longer sailors nor slaves, still they remember
the struck bell piercing sleep, the darkness
below decks where rats splashed in the bilges,
the wide-eyed newborn who flew over the deck rail
saved from the plantation by her mother's arm.

Oceans are thick with them: submariners floating
free of their vaults and pilots whose planes dropped
from the sky like giant guillemots but failed to surface
with a catch of fish. The careless were snatched
by sneaker waves, the joyful by cruising sharks

who dispatched them with a lunge and spat out
their splintered surf boards. Some are surprised
to find themselves here, having thought they'd ascend
to the heaven of upper airs or deep star space. But
these *are* the heavens, say the souls: the heavens below.

John Barton

THE PIANO

It was something you would never let me play, the body
of its music never to be drawn out by my fingers, its keys

tantalizing and just beyond reach, sheet music open on a stand
notes dark as the sheen of its hinged lid, a rich and luminous

eggplant dozing past twilight in a garden you kept to yourself
this upright locked in the study, its body reserved for your touch

alone with it, a test pilot snug inside the cockpit of your Phantom
—you fathered me after the war—such a night fighter high above

us all, high above our dreaming city, speed and ascent scored
across the clouds' wind-shred staff—what bruises, what passion

leafing out, vines climbing into indigo skies, the unpicked glories
of your music camouflaged by the operatic drone of its engines.

John Barton

WARHOL

with apologies to Wayne Koestenbaum

hey there, Drella, it's me, Juan Baton: I erase you; I make you
    live—
the rod I rule with, diseased but social; its potency, prior to
    factory recall

an inflatable function of my body stilled, a balloon subtitling
    the freeze
framed, yawning torture of your films, my screen test becoming
    butcher

with time more shaved and tasty, a beefy snuff movie I am
    starring in
drugged-up, dazed, and odalesque, my cock a colostomy bag
    worn full

frontal and voiding desire, my insides all over your outsides, a
    loudspeaker
between my legs narrating blow jobs, no longer a microphone
    sucking

up passé modernist inhibition as it might have once, genteel and
    hidden
love then allegorical, asexual, allusive, now A-list, aphrodisiac,
    aphoristic

though, unlike you, I remain unAmerican, a foreign body, my
    ambivalent
alien destinies manifestly suspect and pissed away, but, hey, did
    I tell you

I aspire to baldness—so omega, so B-film, to be unwigged out
   as you are
not, balling without tears, this kleptomaniac run-on sentence a
   time capsule

boyfriend after boyfriend after boyfriend after boyfriend after
   boyfriend
after boyfriend after boyfriend after boyfriend after boyfriend
   after boy

friend I lay end to end, the unmourned outlines of their flesh a
   compulsive
silk-screened orgy so empty and repetitious only the brillo-box
   scruples

of a museum could contain them—else no one will—longing
   contemporary
and unnarcissistic only in retrospect, the commercial properties
   of legs

and chests made abstract, dreamy citizens gone art-historical,
   devoid of life
RFK assassinated the day after Valerie shot you, his fifteen
   minutes almost

cancelling out you both, her anger no more notorious than your
   shopaholic
instinct to create, cannibalizing anything in sight, your scarred
   body a work

of the imagination I truss up until the lonely end, this breathy
   parasitic line
a film spliced with commas absent from your posthumous
   diaries, my own

angry voice made to slow down syllable by syllable, frame by
  jerky frame
as I project myself across the ready-made screen of your fame,
  ejaculatory

in homo slow-mo, a low-fidelity money shot so orchidaceous
  you organza—
a deadly improvisation you exteriorize stroke-free over my
  cropped-out face

Bruce Beasley

IDAHO COMPLINE

West, and west, the seeable world
urges, and you're drawn
there too, deviable: quarter-
lit over the half-snag
ponderosa pine, then
glinting under the silt
loam and shale, inside
fire-scarred root-wads
ripped out
of eroded hills . . .

I have to squint
hard to find you
in the dusk shoving the visible lake
back to its far cove;
I have to squint hard
to witness
anything but you
in what dwindles and flames nearby

in the forest understory, where all
is infestation and fight:
crumble of humus,
worm and moss, cancerroot
and skullcap, dwarf
mistletoe deforming the firs
into a gnarl of witches' broom,
unhealable limb—

I glimpse you
rising off the burnt end
of Lost Man Trail, blear
as the drift of mist
into the gulch under Cougar Mountain
where I can't
reassemble you, running
my finger through woodpecker drills
over loose, bug-ridden bark.

There's nothing I want
you to give me:
I've quit asking
for anything but desire—
windflower and anemone in the nurselog's
woodrot.
Everything's gotten out,

Lord,
constellations
dropped like waterstriders on the lake—

What's to come
migrates here in its own time, unhinted-at,
self-divesting

—as you divest
yourself again of all my goings-on,
even the words on my tongue,
the eye as it scans
the blacked-out lake
of Coeur d'Alene,
looking for some sign

of all this signlessness . . .

Bruce Beasley

SELF-PORTRAIT IN INK

As the gone-
translucent

octopus
jet-blasts into evasion, vanishing

while its ink-sac spurts
a cloud of defensive

mucus & coagulant
azure-black pigment,

self-shaped
octopus imago in ink, so the shark

gnashes at that blobbed
sepia phantom,

pseudomorph
that disperses into black

nebulae & shreds
with each shark-strike

& the escaped
octopus throbs

beyond, see-through
in the see-through water, untouched— :

so, go
little poem, little

ink-smudge-on-fingertip
& -print, mimicker

& camouflage,
self-getaway, cloud-

scribble, write
out my dissipating

name on the water,
emptied sac of self-illusive ink . . .

Marvin Bell

PEOPLE WALKING IN FOG

They try to watch themselves, drifting in a white sigh,
the boats and trees, and themselves, too,
when they think of it, spun from sheets of gauzy droplets
with which to tar the morning white and walk upon it.
The horizon yawns. The earth is liquid. They can feel
it, and not just it but the blanket meaning of it.
Here, bravado is the pretense of the immortal
before the infinite. There being no other side,
they must surrender to *this*, seeing they cannot
see far, find a door, hack a hole, or mark a spot.
Goats love fog. Parked lovers and beachcombers
love fog, and those who fear the authorities,
and the camera-shy love it, and they adore it
who wish to be wrapped in beauty so delicate
one must step outside it to be able to see it.

Marvin Bell

"WHY DO YOU STAY UP SO LATE?"

Late at night, I no longer speak for effect.
I speak the truth without the niceties.
I am hundreds of years old but do not know how many
   hundreds.
The person I was does not know me.
The young poets, with their reenactments of the senses, are
   asleep.
I am myself asleep at the outer reaches.
I have lain down in the snow without stepping outside.
I am frozen on the white page.
Then it happens, a spark somewhere, a light through the ice.
The snow melts, there appear fields threaded with grain.
The blue moon blue sky returns, that heralded night.
How earthly the convenience of time.
I am possible.
I have in me the last unanswered question.
Yes, there are walls, and water stains on the ceiling.
Yes, there is energy running through the wires.
And yes, I grow colder as I write of the sun rising.
This is not the story, the skin paling and a body folded over a
   table.
If I die here they will say I died writing.
Never mind the long day that now shrinks backward.
I crumple the light and toss it into the wastebasket.
I pull down the moon and place it in a drawer.
A bitter wind of new winter drags the dew eastward.
I dig in my heels.

James Bertolino

GROWN MEN

Out on the street,
I see two grown men

looking into a tree,
then talking quietly,

eyes cast low. I feel concern,
though I know nothing, have

no reason for this emotion
swelling in me.

Linda Bierds

LAUTREC

Often I fished with my cormorant, Tom,
who would, through wing dips and shudders, identify
the schools. I remember the knots
on his tepid legs, where skin rippled up from the bone,
and the parallel pickets of his shoulders—
how their pivots found echoes
in my knuckles, when I plucked from the sleeve
a granule of ash.

The figure is all, and the figure in motion.

When I opened the fish there were glimmers of
roe, which in turn I turned over
in my study of English: to the deer,
and some dark blemish in mahogany,
in the spill of its quartersawed grain.
How wind through the lips can create such a trio:
fish egg, and doe, and a dapple in wood!

From birth,
my legs held the pliancy of glass.
And shattered, finally, reducing my life to a hobble.
As a boy, rising up from a low chair, I felt
a shin bone buckle and split—a pain,
I assume, like the flare a mollusk must feel, dropped
in the boiling soup. Then the stunned mouth,
all in one motion, closing and opening.

As I fell, I saw in the polished grain of the table
the static figure: roe.

When I was insane, I earned my release
with a family of paintings. A circus. From memory.
Demanded from memory. *As if the functioning mind
is one that imagines.* There were gymnasts
and scarves. And once, on their sides
in a center ring, a woman and horse.

They lay facing each other like lovers, or
the twin lobes of the heart. At the sound of a whistle
each would roll over, roll away, the delicate
legs of the horse flailing a little, stroking the air,
the great body below gathering, shifting,
as a galaxy shifts in its black cabin.
Just before they turned over, each
to a separate world, there is a moment
captured in my painting, an instant,

when the shoe of the woman—its cloud of taffeta bow—
reaches out to the answering hoof of the horse.
Her foot—then, in the distance of
reflection, his: as if he, in some fashion,
were her magnificent extension,
and gave to her eyes what my cormorant saw,
as he entered himself in the passing waters.

Linda Bierds

MEMENTO OF THE HOURS

First the path stones, then the shadow,
then, in a circuit of gorse and mint,
the room with a brook running under it.
It freshened the milk, the cream that grew
in its flat habit a shallow lacquer,
a veil I tested on slow afternoons
with a speckle of pepper.

There was butter, cheddar, the waxy pleats
of squash, green as a storm pond.
Walnuts. Three families of apple,
each with its circle of core fringe.
And the sheen on the walls
was perpetual, like the sheen
on the human body.

My mother would sit with me there,
her draw-string reticule
convex with scent jars and marzipan, the burled
shapes of the hidden. Once she brought her cut
flowers to chill until evening, and told me
the mouths of the bluebells
gave from their nectar a syrup elixir.

It holds in suspension the voices of choirboys,
she said. A dram of postponement.
And I felt as she spoke their presence
among us: the hum
of the brook just under our feet,
the mineral hush of the plenitude,
then the blackened robes of the blackberry vines
gradually filling the door.

Linda Bierds

SHAWL: DOROTHY WORDSWORTH AT EIGHTY

Any strong emotion tempers my madnesses.
The death of beloveds. William in his fever-coat.
I reenter the world through a shallow door
and linger within it, conversations returning,
the lateral cycle of days.

I do not know what it is that removes me,
or sets me again at our long table, two crescents
of pike on a dark plate. But memory lives then,
and clarity. Near my back once again,
our room with a brook at the baseworks,
its stasis of butter and chesse. Or there,

in a corner, my shawl of wayside flowers.
Orchis and chickory. Little tongues of birth-wort.

I remember a cluster of autumn pike
and a dark angler on the slope of the weir.
The fish in his hand and the roiling water
brought forth with their brightness
his leggings and waist. But his torso was lost
into shadow, and only his pipe smoke survived,
lifting, then doubling, on the placid water above him.

Often, I think, I encompass a similar shadow.

But rise through it, as our looped initials
once rose over dye-stained eggs.
We were children. With the milk of a burning candle
we stroked our letters to the hollowed shells.
And dipped them, then, in a blackberry bath,
until the script of us surfaced,
pale, independent, the *D* and cantering *W*,

Then *C* for Christopher. *V*—William laughed—for vale.
And *P*, he said, for Pisces, Polaris, the gimbaling
planets. And for plenitude, perhaps,
each season, each voice in its furrow of air . . .

Once, I was told of a sharp-shinned hawk
who pursued the reflection of its fleeing prey
through three striations of greenhouse windows:
the arrow of its body cracking first into anteroom,
then desert, then the thick mist
of the fuchias. It lay in a bloodshawl
of ruby flowers, while the petals of glass
on the brick-work floor repeated its image.
Again and again and again.
As all we have passed through sustains us.

Linda Bierds

THE THREE TREES

Late day. A wash of claret at the window.
And the room swells with the odor of quince,
tin-sharp and dank, as the acid creeps down
through the etch marks. He dips the foreground languidly,
Rembrandt, so thickets will darken, the horse
and lovers resting there, the bamboo latitude
of fishing pole, the shadowed river.

Then inks it all—mixed sky, three dappled trees—
and presses the intricate net of it
to the white-bleached etching sheet below: one skein
of storm aligning the nothingness, one haycart
rich with villagers. At the window now,

a fading to ochre. And beyond,
through the streets and valley, at the base
of a hillock thick with three trees, a hunter
is ringing a treble bell, its quick bite
driving the field birds to the sheltering grasses.
Around him, dark in their earth-colored clothes,
others are throwing a slack-weave net

out over the meadow and scuttering birds.
And up from their various hands, quick fires bloom,
rush through the beard grass, the birds bursting up
to the capturing net, some dying of fright,
some of flames, some snuffed by the hunters

like candles. A breeze begins, slips through the tree limbs.
Slung over each hunter are threadings of birds,
strung through the underbeak. Pleat-works of plenitude,
down the back, the curve of the shoulder.
They offer their warmth in slender lines,
as sunlight might, through the mismatched shutters
of a great room, the long gaps casting

their cross-hatch. As if time itself might spin them all
down some vast, irreversible pathway—
haycart, hunter, small bowl with its blossoms of quince—
and the simple patterns resting there
barred everything back from the spinning.

Linda Bierds

VAN LEEUWENHOEK, 1675

All day, the cooper's hoops squeal and nibble.
Through the single eyepiece of his hand-ground lens,
he watches a spider's spinnerets, then the tail-strokes
of spermatozoa. Now and then, his bald eye unsquints,
skates blindly across his wrist and sleeve—
and makes from his worlds their reversals:
that of the visible and that of the seen . . .

Visible? he is asked, at the market, or the stone tables
by the river. The lip of the cochineal? Starch
on the membranes of rice? But of course—
though a fashioned glass must press and circle,
tap down, tap down, until that which is, is.

Until that which is, breaks to the eye.
It is much like the purslane, he tells them,
that burst from the hoofbeats of horse soldiers:
black seeds long trapped in their casings, until
the galloping cracked them. In the steppes, he says,

or velt, where nothing in decades had travelled.
Then flowers burst forth from the trauma
of hooftaps, and left in the wake of the soldiers
a ribbon of roadway as wide as their riding.

Smoke now. The screech of a shrinking hoop.
His thoughts are floral with hearth flames and soldiers,
the cords in his bent neck rigid as willow.
Then slowly, below—something yellow. Some flutter of yellow
on the glass plate, in the chamber of a tubal heart . . .

By winter, the snows crossed over the flanks
of the horses, felling them slowly. And the soldiers,
retreating, so close to survival, crept into the bellies
of the fallen bodies. Two nights,
or three, hillocks of entrails steaming like
breath. Now and then they called out
to each other, their spines at the spines
of the long horses, and the flaps of muscle
thick shawls around them. Then they rose, as a thaw
cut a path to the living.

. . . A flutter, yellow, where an insect heart ripples
in reflex. But no, it is only light and shadow, light
turning shadow. As the perfect doors, in their terrible
finitude, open and open.

He straightens, feels his body swell
to the known room. Such vertical journeys, he thinks,
down, then back through the magnifications
of light. And the soldiers, rising, blossoms
of greatcoats on a backdrop of snow:
surely thereafter, having taken through those hours
both the cradle and the grave,
they could enter any arms and sleep.

Anne Caston

HOUSE OF GATHERING

Time blows through and is done.
Those who have come to love him now have
come too late: see how the shadow moves down
at dusk to take the valley
in its arms. Hear the cry
of the corn, wheat whispering

It is time . . .

Listen, he says, *many
children are singing just inside.*
He waves farewell; he enters
alone. The doors shut themselves
after him; the darkness pulls in close.
Only the lights in other houses burn.

Anne Caston

LESSONS FROM THE NATURAL WORLD

Look to the worm.
How well it is made. How
well its mouth accommodates the hook.
Thus hooked, how it complies, how it
takes on the crook and bend
of what runs through it in the end and goes on
writhing, a comely bait—little *come and get me*, little *here am I—*
how you too took on, hard, the shape of your dying.
And while you struggled, crooked, in your bed
Death ran you through from mouth to end
and snapped the thread that held you here.

You're gone. In your absence
how still the water's grown.

Anne Caston

DEPARTURES: LAST FLIGHT FROM FAIRBANKS

Late and we were waiting—sixteen of us—with our coffee
   and carry-ons, impatient for the call to board,
      when a flight attendant appeared, apologizing.

I thought he said he hadn't felt right about sending *ice*
   down the conveyor belt so he'd walked it
      down himself. He placed, on the counter, a box:

insulated, sealed, orange-stickered, all four white sides
   blackly lettered *Human Eyes*. Around the box,
      a hush gathered. Nothing else came near.

Whoever looked at it, looked quickly
   away. When we boarded at last,
      he carried the box

from the terminal, through the dim
   tunnel, onto the bright plane. He held it
      with both hands, in front of him, just inches

from his heart. He watched it in that way
   a child watches what he is told to carry
      carefully: no spilling; no dropping.

I would like to go out like that. I would
   like to be borne one day from this
      body, carried from the black

belly of the beast that mortality is,
   into a last lifting-off. And, before that, I would
      like to wait in some place where a hush gathers

around me one final time
   while the world I have been part of
      goes on as it always has: passing,

impatient, rushing to and fro, terminal
   to terminal, in its long lit
      corridors of sun and moon.

Kevin Craft

HOMEBODY

Tea steeps.
Stones wait.
The status
quo evaporates
like pickets
on a fence.
Only keeps
from going hence
those picaros
at the epileptic gate
dividing prescience
from pretense.

My time has come
and gone,
like a circus
before dawn.
Some say less
is more, others
more or less
derive their loneliness
from plenary session.
I launder
and I laminate.
Who wanders

from task to task
soon founds
a city-state.
One learns
not to mask
long questions.
One counts
on many returns—
as moss
profiles a maple,
as trade winds sop up
oceans ounce by ounce.

Kevin Craft

JANUS-INGENUOUS

January begets journey.
One day is a blue pedestal,
another rushes to meet you
off the ferry with a room to let.

You wouldn't know it
except by the smell of coriander
and the Statue of One Arm
marking the crossroad. Shade

begets shore. Two horn
blasts in the slack water harbor:
arrivals by the bundle,
a packet of farewells.

Only the old, on their mules, stay put.
Or the merchant in the market
weighing mint sprigs green
as the universe seen from a distance.

Or is that latte-beige? Three or four
faces you recognize
but from where? Tomatoes stewing
in their warm red skins.

Forget the annals, the tried tribunes.
Reason is a janitor at the back door
smoking. Yours is the blue door
with the lintel of meat.

There is laundry everywhere
hanging from windows, third
and fourth generation.
Ash begets lather, suds in the harbor.

There are things you should never
forget: God
is a strong detergent.
Look both ways when crossing a sea.

Kevin Craft

TO ERR

It was the era
of ore, of ages ago,
of alps scored by ice
and ill-winds.

It was a Monday
when the month began,
better late
than larvae, better now

than law—it was the eve
of ere too long.
It was what it was,
what it always was,

the aye and awl of it,
the awful arc, the airs.
And yet: I was all ears
beside the sea, mud

in your eye, I was out
of my mind in yon.
It was the era
of *ore*, of italic hours,

walking about
too many urns for a sun.
You were your own
worst enemy, I

the odd one out, ages
of ash ago,
and smoking alps,
and alms.

Kevin Craft

INCENSE

Pungent filament,
            finespun swirling line hung
in air, snaring
            nothing in particular, conspicuous
as a live wire nonetheless:
            how incense
holds sway,
            climbing the narrow chimney of itself
only to
            come undone
at the fluent end
            of its dominion,
giddy as a silkworm gone
            sensationally astray. Here
is the frayed rope charmed out of ash,
            here the nimble
melody of the flute—
            featherweight, aria
of aroma, the air's own
            nom de plume.
Who will trace
            this signature of smolder, who translate
the nomenclature of smell
            as it permeates a room,
path of the supplicant's unhurried prayer?
            Nothing if not
sweet time—sandalwood, scent
            of green mountains, of the redolent
middle of spring—time
            raveling in the deepest sense,
the amnesiac season
            growing fragrant, accountable, as it burns
down the length of its fuse.

Lorna Crozier

ICE-FOG

The air annunciates. It breathes a frosty haze
on my pants and jacket as if I'm growing fur.
Immeasurable, indifferent, now it can be touched
and tasted. It can be seen. Have I fallen through
to the other side of morning or risen above clouds?
This weight, this stillness: splendor thickening.
Down the road a dog barks. Someone walks towards me,
head and shoulders plumed with white. Father?
Lord of Winter? O Death! When his lips touch mine
they will be feathers. I don't know what to do.
I pray for wind, for sun, I pray for my father to speak
before he turns to crystals as he turned to ash.
In the visible around me hoarfrost
hallucinates a thousand shards of bone.

Lorna Crozier

SHADOW

To lie on one side of a tree
then another, over rough or smooth.

To feel cool along one's whole body
lengthening without intent,
nothing getting in the way.

To give up on meaning.
To never wear out or mar.

To move by increments like
a beautiful equation, like the moon
ripening above the golden city.

To be doppelganger,
the feathered underside of wings,
the part of cumulous that slides
thin promises of rain across the wheat.

To disappear. To be blue
simply because snow has fallen
and it's the blue hour of the day.

Lorna Crozier

MELANOMA

The sea keeps coming in,
no one talking. I have to
sit down with the word
for a while. The waves
leave nothing here,
just an upper lip
pinched in the sand
at the highest point.
It keeps on changing.

Many-boned
and maculate, my feet,
one with a scar—
that's what I wanted
to come to—
one with a scar
shaped like a willow leaf.

It glows in the absence
of any light, that other tide
—the dark one—
rolling in.

Lorna Crozier

WALKING INTO THE FUTURE

Months after, your mother's death is
something you pull on every morning,
old flannel tight across your chest.
It's been a hard year—your drinking, stopping,
stopping again, and I've been on the road
too much. Learned a distance I didn't know
before, a space that separates
one phone call, one city from the next. Still,
everything continues, including love,
including loneliness. It's the same
house we live in. Outside, the same tree
splatters our deck with yellow plums,
predictable in late July. Wasps feast
on this sweet mating with the sun.
What changes? Lately there are things
I do not tell you—I ache inside, you
sadden me. Away too long I carry
my bags up the four steps to our porch,
hesitate, as I've never done before.
Sun-blind, I walk into the future,
see only shapes—a couch, a chair,
and someone rising. I don't know who
you will be.

Lorna Crozier

THE NIGHT OF MY CONCEPTION 1

Waiting six years
since my brother drifted from my touch.
I have almost forgotten his smell,
forgotten how we moved together,
water over water, breath riding breath
into the emptiness of blue.

It is the night of my arrival.
My father sits on the couch,
throws a ball for the bull terrier
they've called Patsy.
Behind him my mother bends,
unfastens her stockings.
They slide down her legs
with the sound of sunlight
slipping through the petal of a peony.
Soon he will turn to her.

These are the two
I love and will love
no matter what they do to me
or to each other.
This is my brother's house.

He has opened a window in his room,
the night hot and sticky.
He is trying not to hear
through the wall that keeps him
from the huge bed
they won't let him sleep in any more.

Lightly as a moth I slip
through the screen. He feels
a breeze lifting his hair.
It is me, breathing over him,
savouring his smell,
dusting my small hands
across his forehead
till my mother cries that cry
and I must go.

Months later when he leans
over my crib
he will see it in my eyes,
the way I look at him
as if I know
what he's forgotten

and the first
of the many times
he'll deny me
will begin.

Olena Kalytiak Davis

SHOW UP

at dawn i will rise
to mow my lawn
like the fine young widower
i am

but at dusk i lie still
in the muskeg of my lust
my *i need i want i*
must

and some sometimes one
time time and again lover
busy taken by at
my side

just one time, lover
take me as for what
i am

a not so sleepy not so dreamy
an unreasonable an unseasonable
beauty night can no longer
make right

but my god, what you can awaken to
slaken to rain after so much
sun or vice
verse

each mow row

a year in

a past

a lost

a crossed

a frost covered

a last life

alas life

intact families are all alike
getting into their cars
in raincoats that shine yellow
navy red

thank your dandelion stars
no one is yet is already
dead

lovers, do not come to me
in the dark arrive in the unreal
sidelight of the sidereal
day

pull back your tree covered
curtains to what this world did is
doing while you were down
gone

alas life

at last life

under the nimble limbo of the nimbo
stratus and sphere
right here

in the short torn negligé of my self
-neglect -respect and my wreaking
gortex sneakers

i will have finally shorn
all my scorn then some
fine morn let the line
form:

let all my loves and lovers have the courage to show up
show me what i was worth on this shooting sky green earth

48

Olena Kalytiak Davis

(AND MORE)

(o (l)uxu/orious (p)/(l)ussuria) one can rule
rimini and still not rule (or rim) me. doric, ionic,
phallic: i liked it all. i moaned and wept as i do now,
but it was a joy and a different kind of sorrow:
to see your lover's eyes when he's down there. down there
the very root was the very root, and fig was fruit and nut
gelato. down here how it happened can still make me shudder.
sigh.
just how far down, sinner, must you go? whatever pleases you:
follow my tail, my thigh. and: VIDE FICA MIA. eat my
    furbellowed
heart, tremble at my furbo and my body gone but still beautiful
heart, this life that's for the birds is saved by rhyming such as our
heart, if you twist my arm just right i'll loose my mind.

the new style is the old style: from behind.

Olena Kalytiak Davis

FRANCESCA CAN TOO STOP THINKING ABOUT SEX,
REFLECT UPON HER POSITION IN POETRY,
WRITE A REAL SONNET

pilgrim, i did not mean to be so loose
of tongue, so bold in all i loosely told
in my smut so smug, so overly sold.
i did not mean, pligrim, to traduce.

i apologize, i offer no excuse:
but, poet, though you have right to scold
it was highsouled you who made my mouth hold
what it held and tell what it told. a truce,

no, let's call it an honor. mine is apt,
as far as long sentences go: my vice
in your verse will tempt others to try

and sing: readers, lovers forever rapt
and about to sweetly sigh: paradise!
thank you, poet, for keeping me alive.

Madeline DeFrees

"AFTER GREAT PAIN, A FORMAL FEELING COMES"

It wasn't formal exactly. More like a hummingbird
in the midst of a crow convention: black
cries so raucous they seemed a mockery of common
speech. And the hummer's ultrasonic
whir: wings going nowhere

        over the hearts of flowers,
hovering. What's more, the pain may have been
less than great because it was mainly
physical, the lot of one, not ruby-throated, but
undeniably in the pink.

      Now I cast my fate with
that of the world's smallest bird, impaled on a
purple thistle. With peril every way I turn, and
prone to accident, I earn my
badge of courage diving at eagles, those colossal

birds of prey, deadly as picture windows. Along
the way, my song is mouselike
squeaks, the drone of wings in flight. My heart
like the heart of the hummingbird
equals 20 percent of my weight.

      Day after wrenching
day, I contemplate death, linger over Baltimore
orioles, big frogs, tropical
spiders whose insects feed my hunger. The spider-
silk I wrap around my nest, I ornament with lichen.

Windswept into the river, the current taking over,
I could drown. But I have work to do,
must join the hummingbird to go the distance. Among
the large diurnal fowl—hawks, vultures,
and kites—flight patterns are silhouettes soaring

overhead. Canada geese migrate in formal V's. Like
the hummer, I fill my small crop
with nectar and hope to take my leave mining
the deepest cup in the floral kingdom: red
throat of the trumpet creeper.

Alice Derry

PRECARIOUS

    —John Singer Sargent

Jews as celebration.

One daughter, you made Turkish musician,
one, gypsy holding a broomstick.
More than one in red, lips bright,
eyes daring any of us
to get a life.

Mrs. G's shoulder strap.
After you'd ingratiated yourself with her.
She just as attracted.
Of course it cost you ground with the rich,
probably *because* she was cheating on her husband.

Money and power.
But your clients didn't trust the camera—so lately come to
   them.
They depended on you.

Who could resist *not* giving them what they hungered for?

Still, you didn't rub their faces in the life-sized male nudes
I'm spending time on:
nude after nude after nude.
Giving myself my obligatory twenty minutes getting over that
   many genitals
that baldly hung,
I'm overcome by the sweet exuberance of the bodies,
how tenderly vulnerable,
how you *use* them, sprawled in every compromising pose,
voyeurism
lust.

"Was he a lover of women?" Bernard Berenson's asking (archly)
   as late as 1957.
Oh, come on.

You kept the glittering black girl from Crete
for your own collection.

You turned the body of the black man Thomas E. McKellar
into a Greek god in the Boston library murals.
But I doubt if you were thumbing your nose at secret racism.
It's clear you'd fallen in love with a shape,
as one might fall in love with rolling hills,

you'd fallen for a glance.
In the portrait of him as him, he opens his legs in trust,
his eyes hold steady
while his penis lolls to one side.

How often women see it that way—
our eyes caught in the middle of his huge body,
mortified that *human* means
a mind to reason us out of brutal desire—
yet it can't.

What kept you from joining
Monet or Van Gogh, living hand to mouth,
painting exactly what they liked and scorned for it?

After all, you didn't just bring the Wertheimers
daringly close to royal portraiture,
acknowledging, taunting.
You let the family invite you over for supper,
sat with them and became friends.

So that nothing I see today is head on
but bears its undeniable
double blade.

You didn't—couldn't?—prevent the youngest
Wertheimer from being detained while singing opera in Italy.
The Nazis killed her.

That later photo of you from 1910, painting outside in
   Switzerland,
gone to fat, mustached. Vest and coat and hat.
You're staid. You've got yourself covered.

Candice Favilla

DO NOT FORGET MY NAME

—for Daria and my sisters

So here's to Rosa Luxembourg
And the unblessed class of working poor,

Who, like a heart at a door,
Expect beauty to open and give more.

Here's to us. Drink up and wait,
Holding our mud and nibbling the bait.

Waiting will give everything. But
The stuff we use for barter

Is mostly gone, mere as the brevity of thought:
We should move on but we cannot.

As though to think were to own a thing,
We're as temporary as the TV's claims. Who knows,

Another month could restore us. Talking.
Talking. His "haves and have mores" walking

Over us while we, in our study of trauma,
Build our lives of factory drama

And brief dolly-fucks in parking lots.
We suspect it's real only

Because it's rough, it makes us feel tough,
and the concrete stinks of piss, gasoline,

And the drunk in his bedding.
I'm pregnant every year: kids smashing

Stick ball in shit-house
Alleys. Look around you,

Everybody knows this story; factory's gone:
Poor Luck got to have

Some children. While old men, shambling
In the parks, mutter how succulent was

A blackberry of the past—
Before we all were losers

And the dollar rose and set—
No good nostalgia in this and nothing

More mysterious than that
At the end of our lives

We'll all cry out for one
More moment in the sweet flesh.

Some call me irreligious.
But I bargained, voted, begged, and prayed.

But was nothing would make the work go easy
When I had no work, when no work gave.

Candice Favilla

SEEDTIME

Rusted silver '60's Valiant wagon
with slant block and dents and the first bucket seats ever
sis's husband chants, even if ripped and valves so blown
and carburetor so crapped out the car merely hiccups up
an incline, merely chuckles so that the Highway 90 overpass
looms large before us with its daunting ramp, fifty feet of
    torment—
will we die crushed beneath truck tires? And we—sis, her three
    babes and I—
we are moving slowly with huge rigs hauling chattel and
    chemical spill
through the western world, trundling past, beating out burps
of beware! On horns threateningly near, fast past us and
    bumping
dusts to semi trucks' furious din. My sister, filter tip
Marlboro peeling off carbon snakes of poison from her left
    hand
as she negotiates some wheel, half turns to slap
with her right at the scrambling kids in the back, who all have
filthy noses and hard candy smears bought at the Disco with
    Welfare,
and we are moving one chug at a time, stinky exhaust
    surrounding
our bearings forth, aura by which anybody might prognosticate
futuromachies in mega-rut or a promise
concerning future success not even a postal worker can miss
a guess at, and I am scrunched low and eleven years old in the
    front seat and searing heat
off the fagged engine competes with that of the summer
landscape of blacktopped suburbs—110 degrees—I watch
    through snot-smeared glass.
Maples, fried flower beds, starched wives below anchored to
    turned-on hoses

and juxtaposed to flat-butted husbands poured beneath Fords
in communal driveways. Slowly the rooftops slide from angled
   to flat as
we falter and climb, and my sister hoorays, "Stop fighting I'll
   kill you," and smacks
the kids, and cigarette smoke and exhaust in a wave nauseates
   our eyes as we slow,
—slow,—rock in the buckets—inchmeal, lollygagging,
   birdbrained—climb
skyward. How long, Lord, how long?

Candice Favilla

CAPITULATIONS

1

They are from hunger, she says. In China her family lost their land, plots of caraway, homes, babies. Many times, to give these up. Cabbages to the government, to have a season's crops replaced by a few allotted bundles of parsley breaks and leeks. You ask them and they say, "Eat bitter."

2

Haldol, white sludge in a plastic cup, cakes at the corners of his mouth, bloats his face. He nods from his bed. Well, now you've made it, odd tyrant, husband. Must I gather you in fragments— My Life My Husband—alone? He weighs less than I, now. I could fling him around the room to visit with the clutch of flowers I plucked from our garden. I can beat him if I wish, while he lies there dumb as our first child, burned stupid in my womb sixty years ago. If he does not insist too violently on his own willful identity, he may live like this for years. In this dingy room. No relief from the buzzing television. Outside, it's April. Look, Old Pencil, Old Drop-cloth, I'd invite you along if you knew I was going. Is there a last time for us you remember? The flesh doesn't; it yellows. Dear-after-the-stroke, I'm your loving menace.

3

The body like a viral strain spills out its deception. It is greedy, this landlord. Fog at a field's edge—that's my brain. Dehydration, bone scrapes bone, each spinal disk clacking like a gun lock when I rise, knee and hip bone seizing in the sockets.—Moving, I clunk like a wind chime: skeleton hung on a windy hill. Quixote gone. Buzzards flapping near. What is more succinct than pain? The 5 cc's of syrupy chemicals mixed in a syringe and injected subcutaneously, hot sickness injected weekly, which is cure. Emboldened fever, itself a journey, the endless bed of twisted dampened sheets, the less and less of me as I lie beneath my eye and watch my muscles melt. Vomit. Brain fevers. Stubborn decay of the muzzy mind: "Distraction with too much representation," the doctor quips. "We call it a cure."

Tess Gallagher

BULL'S-EYE

Driving to the ferry,
that reverie releasing
the unsaid, I tell my friend
it's *okay. I'll be okay.*
When the doctor
said *There's no cure*
an arrow flew out of
the cosmos—*thung!*
Heart's center. Belonging
to everything. That
quick.
                    for Valerie

Tess Gallagher

CHOICES

I go to the mountain side
of the house to cut saplings,
and clear a view to snow
on the mountain. But when I look up,
saw in hand, I see a nest clutched in
the uppermost branches.
I don't cut that one.
I don't cut the others either.
Suddenly, in every tree,
an unseen nest
where a mountain
would be.

for Drago Štambuk

Tess Gallagher

NOT A SPARROW

Just when I think the Buddhists
are wrong and life is not mostly suffering,
I find a dead finch near the feeder.
How sullen, how free of regret, this death
that sinks worlds. I bury her near
the bicycle shed and return to care for
my aged mother, whose suffering
is such oxygen we do not consider it,
meaning life at any point exceeds
the price. A little more. A little more.

That same afternoon, having restored balance,
I discover a junco fallen on its back, beak
to air, rain pelting the prospect. Does
my feeder tempt flight through windows?
And, despite evidence, do some
accomplish it?

Digging a hole for the second bird, I find
the first gone. If I don't think "raccoons"
or "dogs," I can have a quiet, unwitnessed
miracle. Not a feather remains.
In goes the junco. I swipe earth over it,
set a pot on top. Time
to admit the limitations of death as
admonition.

Still, two dead birds in an afternoon
lets strange sky into the mind: birds flying
through windows, flying through
earth. Suffering must be
like that too with inexplicable escapes where the mind
watches the hand level dirt over the emptied grave
and, overpowered by the idea of wings,
keeps right on flying.

WEATHER REPORT

The Romanian poets
under Ceausescu, Liliana
said, would codify opposition

to the despots in this manner: because
there was no gas and they were cold, everyone
was cold, all they had to do was write

how cold it is . . . so cold . . . and their
readers knew exactly what was meant.
No one had to go to jail
for that.

Liliana, in the dead of night
writing her poems
with gloves on.

I think I'll take off my gloves.
It's freezing in here.
There's a glacier pressing on my heart.

Gary Gildner

CLEANING A RAINBOW

I open it with my long blade under the bright flow
of well water and there lie the finny wings
a moth is beginning to fold,
and then I see the river again, and where I stood
in sun- and rain-slant, that arc of color, the trout
coming down, pulling everything with it, the cold mountain
stream, the boulders blue and yellow and red, pines wind-
    pushed
among them and scrubbed to a silvery finish, current-salved,
    their limbs
lashed by tendrils of pale canary grass, all inside it and coming
    down,
the veined pebbles inside it and coming down, rolling, even the
    pearly
stone a raw-throated raven kicked loose, the love-sick bray
a wandering mule gave out causing a moose at first-
light browse to look up, the moony call
an owl still can't stop giving softly inside it, the slow-waking
kayaker's deep satisfying sleep washed from her eyes vividly
    inside it,
all inside it and coming down, finding their places, the
    feathered layers
of flesh making room, the pursy fir and lean young alders
in league with the willows, all bending, their refusals to snap
quietly folded inside it, their needles and leaves and aspirations,
    too
subtle to separate, completely inside it, tracks large and showy
and barely there become petite, hair-thin bones, become
    murmuring
rib-chimes, choirs, echoes from the lightest touch inside it and
    coming
down the river, embraced by the scent of cherry and musk, by
    the shy
fairy slipper, by bear's breath and the must oozing

from a single wild grape, by incense cedar, myrtle
and skittish skunk, all rank and sweet together, all
brushings and sighs coming down, through slick spidery worm-
    scrawl
falling, flicker-knock, locked horn and cocky treble-cry falling,
    famous
stalkings and leaps lost in the furling eddies, the heart sucked
under, fibril and seed and viscid yolk sucked under, necks
nuzzled, licked, whirling around astonished, dogtooth violet
    and thorny
rose bush torn from their root mesh, garnishing all, and
    everyone rushing
down, down to this small washing, this curl of final composure
I hold in the bowl of my hands kneeling to receive it.

68

Gary Gildner

HAPPINESS JAZZ

Okay, that number comes up
with or without much help.
Mothers, brothers, friends, all
kinds of people—kind, cruel,
little kids when you least
expect it—ask for it. First
thing the morning after hard
self-abuse, even you've had
the urge to wish for a bite.
Even old Franklin, the crafty kite
guy, said Hey, wait a minute,
when T.J. wrote *life, liberty,
and the protection of property.*
Said we want the pursuit
of something that juices.
Like sex, like food, like Jesus
and rime, time hasn't put
much of a stop, much of a boot
to its chops. Teeth, baby, it's got
molars, precious metals, fangs,
a grip that won't quit, lungs,
lug nuts, sunsets, dawns dappled
and crippled, shims missing, trouble
in mind, howls, oh no's, new shoes
that slide & glide, sass, the blues
to bring a person around exactly
when he or she's down inexactly.
Come on, B-flat, lift that head so
heavy, that heart so full,
break through and spill
over, way over, honey,
let go and grab hold
as if you had *all* the money.

Gary Gildner

THE GIG

They invited me in, then
asked what I played.
I said horn. They
handed me one with a long cord
hanging down. They said
sample it, man. I
put the small round end
to my mouth and blew—
it was okay. Unusual
but okay. Then the guy
on sax tapped out one, two,
one, two, three and we started.
He was good, he grew large
wings, wings and a deep concern.
Everyone stopped, including me.
The question seemed to be:
where were we?
I felt bad. My timing
was slow, the sound
I pushed out full of
wet air, farty.
And that cord kept
getting underfoot.
But I wasn't going to
make excuses. My horn
was a damn lamp
with a yellow shade.
My lips were sore.
So what? This was the gig.
Let's go, I said. Let's play.

Michele Glazer

SONNET

> *The threatened vernal pool fairy shrimp is a 3/4-inch translucent*
> *crustacean with a one-year life cycle and a unique survival strategy.*

Invisible in vernal pools——

the fairy shrimp have no secrets.

But if their bodies are——in water——

as transparent as desire what

can desire hold?

This close to bodiless——what they possess

they will not have and what's seen-

through seems only there by her

imagining them. So that later

when his fingers touched her navel————*I'll kiss you*

there, only——is what he said and let his mouth roam

up to where the quartermoon of one breast

quieted him, she could feel how he had practiced

this before with his eyes closed   and alone.

Michele Glazer

HISTORIC HOUSE, ASTORIA

I was there for the invention of nostalgia.
It wasn't for everyone and never would be
though the view has changed. Freighters
lining the channel on their way
upriver to the other city, these were the past.
It isn't the room I want but the view from out the window.
The doors and knobs disclose the probably height of the owners
    and
from their bunks at night sailors could smell the trees
from miles off shore. Back then the future was far away
but when you get there
it's just as big as what you left
though some of the details have been lost.
Someone had to go far into the community,
bringing back breadboards all circa the same
until the house is more as we imagine than how it was.
It wasn't my old life I wanted but the one that had eluded me.
I examine the roundness of nooks and mantels.
Side-buttoning white shoes.
The trees are small because the weather's hard
though feet in general have grown in length
and spread over
the past 100 years.

Michele Glazer

MAP

Everywhere there was a bush and a bird in it.
Things popped out of the grasses
clicking and you knew
you were walking in nature, entering Brush Canyon
exiting Bird so I kept thinking why
should I be the one always asking where it hurts?
Somewhere we paused where
a plank got wedged between trees,
tight so we could sit on it. I touched the wound
—that something viscous
could be pitch at an attitude that hard.
Where Bird Canyon was subsumed by Bear Gulch
the one I was with peeled off to shortcut up some shortcut
so I walked up Downey Gulch through a saw of indolent cows.
I knew them for what they were—red eyes, bulk
and jitteriness—
the way it's always something.
For the first time it was clear to me
that the lines on my map were the draws
and gullies I was lost in
so I couldn't stay lost. That night the sky was nothing
but stars and the crickets made a curtain of sound.
Why can't I remember that? He washed my hair.
I lay on the porch with my neck extended; he rested
my head in his open hand. The sky had rounded
up all its citizens and pressed down.

Patricia Goedicke

AT THE EDGES OF EVERYTHING, CRACKLING

In almost tidal movements,
      people crowding together
   back and forth   shifting

looks given   then taken away
        hooks and   uneasy whispers
            trickling out from the faint fringes of things

fiery sun matter   invisible
        sways from one planet
   one shoulder to another

passing each other   cats
      slide through doorways
          in opposite directions tingling   fine hairs   rise

cells heave outwards
        towards other cells   bulging
    at the edges of everything   crackling

exiles hide in the passes
        brandishing their new   cell phones
                armies call across canyons

meteors in space flash
      across the horizon   dit-dotting over helmless
   radioactive fields

oscillant specks   flickering
      in each closed system connected
          somewhere   o far star

Patricia Goedicke

SIX SHORT ONES

Towards the End

When it is still.
When a dog can lie out on it and never look back.
In the wrecked gymnasiums of the mind.
In the very temple of it.

When the paraclete tellers roll over and play dead.
When cars in the distance backfire, when the lakes are frozen over.
In Chicago, granite. Marbled in silent San Francisco.

When moose dream of cities.
When the sky's lid rumbles, the attack planes are heading out.
Is this, then, what it is?
And no casinos to save us.

One Button for the Smoke Jumper

Underwater drowned eyes. Heavy gelatin on the neck, buttoned
    in topaz
but duller, bottled and jailed sunglasses not. As weird amber
    oblonged, hard hemmed and egg yolked to no air or little.
    Pinpricks, choked and rasped mufflers of no fire
but smoked oceans, barrelfuls of it no one can rowboat through
    but rubbery,
on sizzling apricot boots sideways.

Cheap

Yesterday drinking too much cheap white wine,
today a copper red Irish Setter comes swimming —
long nose gentlemanly, sleek as a yacht's prow,
steady as a Cambridge lady's bicycle on a straight path
over four feet pedaling gently, in the clear green underneath —
eyes filling with tears again: too many blue skies, brief showers,
  gray sunshine.

Adventures of a Lost Buddha

Footsteps walk the drive, an elderly frog hops into the garage. What happened to the key? And where do we keep the nerve gas? She keeps looking for it. Vague whiffs of it seep everywhere. Rainbows hiss in her ears. But everyone said she should wake up, play Handel's Fireworks. Several others were waiting in the livingroom, miowing. To Piazzola and a couple of blondes slinking their mean tangos. Yes there was a Bush in the outhouse. Donkey thighs for the unwary. How unpolitic. Death, thou art a pruned swan, little black seed in the corner. Very felt, very feelingful. Teeth stuck together by bubble gum. Friendly, he brought them out, police dogs in a back alley. As the puppet masters perch in the rafters, weep crocodile rivers for the children. This is his amphitheater, so what if he blows it up. All of it.

At a Later Party

She said they were crying together, the three friends at the party, sitting together in a corner.

She said they were crying together, talking about the disease that had come back for one of them for good.

She didn't say what it was like, this crying?
She didn't have to.

Pistachios

Finally the woman feels like an old tree trunk, toppled. Grubs walk around in her stomach, she sleeps. But she's cold. Her extremities are freezing. Her sick ivory index, her third and fourth fingers. Whenever the cold at her heart, the wind off the mountains . . . . Her bed is narrow, she thinks she is dying: everyone is dying. While she's still living! Things are happening to her, she knows that. Perhaps she is only living more deeply? It's amazing how many strange ideas come to her everyday. Pistachios falling out of a bag whenever you try to close it. But she is tired sometimes, too tired, and many of her branches ache. Tuning forks tingle and buzz shockingly, *Zing!* So she moves slowly. Though the pistachios keep coming, each morning a new one. Some beautiful, popped open overnight. Who will take care of them when she dies. Who will eat them.

Patricia Goedicke

THE QUESTION ON THE FLOOR

Some mornings the body wakes to itself
                    as to an ocean, the soft wash of it
        on a shore it wants to love. Lie back, love, it says,
                            and let me lift you,
            the sheets touching you are waves,
    are the cool shock of first sun over the mountain lighting
                the ceiling, then the floor—Ah yes, the floor

the body says to itself, those skeleton boards
                        that trip. Splinter. Stumble us
            to our knock knees backhanded—

But is this proper, is it mete?
            Especially after the calm. The miraculous
                    svelte peace of the sea, say, after lovemaking
            which never lasts, Horatio, which never lasts—

Though waves of liquid salt lap at each other, circulating
    around the world
            this tidal lymph (which is everywhere) is a mess
                    of needy corpuscles unmoored,
                free form. Floating.

As the great capricious Body above us moves (regretfully) on,
                    the question, still on the floor,
            is a tongue of greasewood burning
                        to answer itself,
                to contain its own dissolving
        in little permanent cups:
                    snapshots

of what we used to look like: what cells
                                    eventually consumed us
and what we cooked for the picnic, what blessings, how many
    oysters,
        pink slabs of salmon on the grill entered and then left us—
                        Or pancakes, for the last time
                    or kisses (which are words)

and more kisses, and more—
            as the entire shore line falls away out from under us,
        the diamond polished grit of the great sand dunes,
                                their chewed driftwood,
            their ground up shells collapsing
                until all our secret interiors, our separate identities,
        all bits and pieces of us are no more.

James Grabill

WHEN KALI DANCES THE EARTH AROUND

Through the nuthatch's eye, we saw spaces
between branches and leaves
that molecules have and cells use for breathing.
We stood up in the dome of the cherry,
and it was setting sun striking towering trees in the east.
Blazing infiltrated to coach regular formation,
charged by nuclear seeds, nuclear hair, telephone sky,
nuclear bread, chanted in atomic sparrow song
upsurged by wind threading days onto chains of months,
months into months, months into centuries, beaded
as blue earth stones one after the other in a bracelet
Kali wears on one of her wrists, a skull housing each stone
in the shadow of the bank complex towering here, not here,
here, not here with belching Motorola of Mercury
loosened into waters, soaked up by the fish we've eaten,
crimson sublunar chords in this neighborhood Milky Way.

We sat back into spaces splendorized by army personnel
whose eyebrows hang with long Pacific rainforest
moss over our words, our pittance swallowed
by ocean when we dropped a human anchor
of forgiving that was suffering what could only be
our ignorance. Many suns had been out, in vast expanses,
beyond thinking, the certain answers out with them,
beading month after month, months into century
after century into Kali's anklet rocked
when the planet grows round.
Now black forests turn hot and blazing in the heart of the sun.

Neile Graham

THE WALK SHE TAKES

—Smailholm Tower, the Border Country—

Slow in the weight of the fog
on the rolling lands of the Merse—green, green
old hills—she hears the steps of ghost horses,
echoing hooves and rain.

In this distance where there is no distance
all horses are ghosts,
all wind the lament of the border widow,
she:
   "I took his body on my back and whiles I gaed,
   and whiles I sat, I digged a grave and laid him in
   And happ'd him up with sod sae green.'

Walking she traces the furrowed line
of a runrig—lines
that disappear underfoot. Lines
of cottage walls
leaning up against the laird's protection.
She can step right over the barmkin now, so little
of its height remains,

step in and out of strangers' lives: the old lord
who lost three brothers and a son at Flodden,
then the years after staggered by the reivers
stealing first 600 cattle then 123 then 60 then 6,
100 prisoners taken then 4.

It's here she finds her man leaning against a wall
of this tower brittle-patched with memories
patterned with blood and fear rising above the earth
into fog woven with wraiths and lamentations

crumbling alone. She's walking the borders,
she's out ghosting. She's getting used to harm.

Neile Graham

GRAVES AND CHURCHYARDS CAIRNS AND CAIRNS

By whom the subterraneous vaults are peopled is now utterly unknown.
The graves are very numerous, and some of them undoubtedly contain the
remains of men, who did not expect to be so soon forgotten.
        —from Samuel Johnson's A Journey to the Western
            Isles of Scotland *(1775)*

the afterlife alive under stone
peopled by shadows skulls unruly dust
as we exploring exploit the world underground
tourists in cairns souterrains tombs

peopled by shadows skulls unruly dust
the bones of eagles deer and dogs
tourists in cairns souterrains tombs
their age measured in thousands of years

the bones of eagles deer and dogs
add fleetness to the weight of human remains
their age measured in thousands of years
counted in hundreds under the nearby church floor

add fleetness to the weight of human remains
the walls rise over them blocks of stone
counted in hundreds under the nearby church floor
someone rests beneath the stones beneath our feet

the walls rise over them blocks of stone
each bone placed by human hands
someone rests beneath the stones beneath our feet
and the flesh that nets our bones is thin

each bone placed by human hands
we are the gravid robbers of graves
and the flesh that nets our bones is thin
we belong here by our presence alone

we are the gravid robbers of graves
as we exploring exploit the world underground
we belong here by our presence alone
the afterlife alive under stone

Catherine Greenwood

TWO BLUE ELEPHANTS

I
Two elephants: blue as sky absorbed
in bodies of water, vessels of grief
so ancient they merely grin,
the marrow in their spongy bones sorrow,

blink from the glazed stones of their eyes
salt sweated from centuries of drought,
raise trunks to scout moisture,
shake dirt from cracked hides and hoist themselves,
huge sacks of tears, up on wrinkled knees.

From the sediment of a sea-bed
gone arid, they rise in a mist of dust
and begin to batter wearily a door
rusted shut, portal to the barnacled heart
of a hold filled with a fortune in sand dollars.

II
Can you not feel it, the world
shudder and tremble as it strains
against its hinges? We are lost
as gods who've lumbered into the wrong continent
and, without solace of worship, look down
to find their broad feet fashioned
into umbrella stands. How futile
the parasols we so foolishly pitch
against pain, as if it were as simple
as believing, as repelling sun or rain.

Here, I'm breaking this blue sleeping
tablet in two and sending you half
that together we may fall
into a slumber and wake
on either side of the same dream.

Lord of Doorways,
accept our simple offering:
the turquoise mirror in a mountain lake,
sesame cake baked with seed
stolen from the hidden cave,
mouse milk thinned with evaporated tears.

Open, let us in.

John Haines

POEM FOR THE END OF THE CENTURY

I am the dreamer who remains
when all the dreams are gone,
scattered by the millennial winds
and sacked by the roadside.

The solar clockhand stopped,
confusion and fury on the street
—so much idle paper
shredded and tossed aside.

The small, dim shops of the tourist
trade are shuttered and locked . . .
Nightfall, and the buyer turns away.

One more stolen fortune spent,
another century gone
with its fits and desolations—
I leave my house to the creditor wind.

Tell me if you know my name,
whose face I wear, whose stored-up
anger fades to a tentative smile.

I am the one who touches fire,
who rakes the leaves to watch them burn,
and who says once more to himself
on this calm evening of earth:

Awake! The stars are out,
mist is on the water,
and tomorrow the sun will return.

1999

John Haines

THE LEGEND

I.

I understand the story of Gilgamesh,
of Enkidu, who called the wind by name,
who drank at the pool of silence,
kneeling in the sunburnt shallows
with all four-footed creatures.

I know the name of that exile,
the form that it takes within us:
the parting and breaking of things,
the distance and anguish.

I know, too, in its utter strangeness,
that whoever asks of the sun its rising,
of the night its moonstruck depths,
stirs the envy of God in his lofty cabin.

And when Enkidu awoke, called
from his changed, companionless sleep
—singly, in glittering pairs,
the beasts vanished from the spring.

II.

The forest bond is broken,
and the tongued leaves no longer
speak for the dumb soul lost
in the wilderness of his own flesh.

All that had life for him:
the moon with her wandering children,
the storm-horse and the shepherd-bird,
become as salt to his outspread hand.

Let him go forth, to try the roads,
become that wasted pilgrim, familiar
with dust, dry chirps and whispers;
to die many times—die as a man dies,
seeing death in the life of things.

And then descend, deep into rootland
—not as a temple-gardener, planting
with laurel the graves of gods and heroes,
but as one grieving and lost . . .

To ask of the dead, of their fallen
web-faces, the spider's truth,
the rove-beetles's code of conduct.

By such knowledge is he cured,
and lives to face the sun at evening,
marked by the redness of clay,
the whiteness of ash on his body.

III.
By stealth, by the mastery of names,
and one resounding axe-blow
rung on the cedar-post at dawn,
the great, stomping bull of the forest
was slain. Rain only speaks
there now on the pelted leaves.

Overheard through the downpour,
in the stillness of my own
late-learned solace, I understand
through what repeated error
we were driven from Paradise.
The nailed gate and the fiery angel
are true.
      Could we ask them,
speaking their wind-language
of cries, of indecipherable song,
it may be that the swallows
who thread the water at evening
would tell us; or that the sparrows
who flock after rain, would write
in the coarse yellow meal
we have strewn at the threshold,
why God gave death to men,
keeping life for himself.

For the strong man driven to question,
and for him who, equally strong,
believes without asking,
sleep follows like a lasting shadow.

1981–1996

John Haines

FOR THE HOMESTEAD FRIENDS

—after Horace

Our bottle of malt is nearly drained,
our stories are told, our poems
remembered and recited. Now the woodland
ghosts return to be our witness.

We have walked the trails I cleared
forty-five years ago, and cleared
again when I returned to claim
my house and land too long neglected.

I see the blaze-marks, still yellow
in the bark of the trees I spared.
I see the fallen fence-posts of a garden
long kept, now gone to mice and weeds.

Where are the men who settled here,
who named the creeks and hills,
and made of that their hometown legend?
I feel an absence in the summer light.

Campbell with his dogs on Buckeye,
that long last mile uphill; Doherty,
a good man far from Ireland, and
Issacson—the names so easily lost.

Who was it built the cabin I moved
and saved? —His lonely life and death
before I came, long buried now
at Birch Hill under a lettered stone.

And Melvin, at eighty-six, still active
with his last moose down and he alone
to do that work . . . I hear his voice,
his hand steady at the roadhouse table.

And we who sit here now, companions
in the making of another story
to be told, perhaps, one far-off
August evening in this very room.

We've had a day . . . Then sleep, think
of the morning to come, and all
that we can do or hope to do, before
this fading summer turns to frost.

Be still. One final toast to friends
who are not here, remembered neighbors.
And read, if you will, or speak,
one poem appropriate to the night.

1999–2000

Kathleen Halme III

COMB

Perhaps I was naïve. I thought it was for beauty:
the bees' stacking their bits of wax
in vertical combs as lattices of six.
The Honeycomb Conjecture now holds this shape
is the most economical partition of a plane
into equal areas and uses the least wax to form
built-ins—the honey, pollen, larvae bins. We know that
bees have three tasks: food, dwelling, toil;
and the food is not the same as the wax,
nor the honey, nor the dwelling.

Did you know you can train honey bees
to come to cardboard flowers?
After you cut out the flower shape you must
place a bottle cap of sugar water in the flower's center.
Pulled to hive, syrup-loaded,
bees tell bees how to find the flowers.

On my desk I keep a cake of beeswax, palm-size
polygon, six-sided, impressed with tiny hexagons,
a six-legged bee raised in the center,
wings folded like a membrane cloaked
in spice of midday beam through leaf.

I smell it every day for faith.
I bought it from a drowsy farm boy yawning
over a glass suitcase of bees working
on their comb. I, too, am an artificer and felt close.
Pure beeswax, it says,
(go in fear of quasivatic drones).

Form of form of form. Sure, it's pure—
wax, wholly wax, yet it mimics maker
and made. It leaves no space.
What if butter came shaped as an udder?
Clumsy jilter of maker and made,
it leaves no space.

I've tried to make way for myth,
but this longing for shapes
as elegant as instinct persists.

Kathleen Halme III

DRIFT AND PULSE

Her moon   opens
to   your moon
a pumping   shadow
of heart   no heart
a haloform   an oblate I
underfrilled
in crinolines   a ballgown's
sway   and slave
in champagne stockings
Out of her
element   she is
an apostasy   on paper
eggwhite smear
in a library   book
pulsing iambs   oral arms
fleshpot shadow   of heart   no heart
see   through soul
in plexiglass   No brain   no bones
no spine   no heart
form's form

Kathleen Halme III

WHAT SELF

Nothing lived on land, nothing had
crawled out of the shallow sea.

Because they have no hard parts,
it's rare to find the fossil of a jelly.
The farm boy digging a new duck pond
exposed thousands, like old verbs
stranded on the shore of the lonely
Paleozoic; nothing came to eat them,

nothing was sloshing in the shrimpdom.
A see-through diving bell as formal as a ghost,
the giant medusa waved her oral arms to subtilize her food.
Who said life unfolds in language?

Nothing lived on land, nothing had
crawled out of the shallow sea.

Sam Hamill

LESSONS FROM THIEVES

1.
Someone has stolen my orchid—
nothing left but a circle
of emptiness in the dust.

Alas. Alas, goddammit.
I loved that flower too much.

2.
Was it the flower I loved,
or only the intricate
nurturing and the patience?

Winter solstice is over.
Soon the camellia will bloom.

3.
What you have taken from me
is merely your illusion.
What is mine cannot be yours

because you cannot grasp it—
no questions and no answers.

4.
Here is the Buddha's flower.
Is it his or is it yours?
The flower is your teacher

or your product, your emblem—
a dragon is in your fist.

5.
I'll cherish this emptiness
you left behind. "Attain *hsu*!"—
Lao Tzu—"Emptiness supreme."

The flower is in the pot.
The blossom is in the mind.

Sam Hamill

THE NEW YORK POEM

I sit in the dark, not brooding
exactly, not waiting for the dawn
that is just beginning, at six-twenty-one,
in gray October light behind the trees.
I sit, breathing, mind turning on its wheel.

Hayden writes, "What use is poetry
in times like these?" And I suppose
I understand when he says, "A poet
simply cannot comprehend
any meaning in such slaughter."

Nevertheless, in the grip of horror,
I turn to poetry, not prose,
to help me come to terms—
such as can be— with the lies, murders
and breathtaking hypocrisies

of those who would lead a nation
or a church. "What use is poetry?"
I sat down September twelfth,
two-thousand-one in the Common Era,
and read Rumi and kissed the ground.

And now that millions starve
in the name of holy war? Every war
is holy. It is the same pathetic story
from which we derive
"biblical proportion."

I hear Pilate's footsteps ring
on cobblestone, the voice of Joe McCarthy
cursing in the senate, Fat Boy exploding
as the whole sky shudders.
In New York City, the crashes

and subsequent collapses
created seismic waves. To begin to speak
of the dead, of the dying . . . how
can a poet speak of proportion any more
at all? Yet as the old Greek said,

"We walk on the faces of the dead."
The dark fall sky grows blue.
Alone among ash and bones and ruins,
Tu Fu and Basho write the poem.
The last trace of blind rage fades

and a mute sadness settles in,
like dust, for the long, long haul. But if
I do not get up and sing,
if I do not get up and dance again,
the savages will win.

I'll kiss the sword that kills me if I must.

Jerry Harp

A DAY LIKE THIS

This guy approached me at the mall.
He had eyes like nuclear fission.
He said, "The universe is a long division

of aromatic astral projections.
My wife channels the great teachers.
You see, we're metaphysicians."

Then he did a kind of dance,
a shuffle to the side and a hop.
He tried to decipher my hairline,

but my head's an illegible scrawl,
so he took off his shirt and pants.
I said, "I'm only here to buy some paint.

I haven't been current for years,
though I do have a volume at home
written by a medieval saint.

We moved in a dance across the floor,
our hands coordinated with precision.
Was that music coming from a star?

I wrote Vita Nuova on his hip.
A woman in light held a book
and improvised koans in Greek

as she ascended beyond the coffee nook.
My friend did legerdemain with being and seem.
We'd become a metaphysical team.

Jerry Harp

THE CREATURE QUOTIDIAN

Lie down at the fringe of a nightmare—
Its enclosures and swamps, a friendly place
After all, made kinder by the utter indifference
Of every face on the train taking us into the woods
Where snakes on the rocks catch some sun.

The city lights loom up, jewels in the mud.
Day and night I pedal past the banks,
The schools, the repairmen, and the nuns.
I've forgotten my destination, though I need
No destination, only concrete, sand, and sun.

The syllables that circulate like blood
Through every node and mode of consciousness
Never could quite cohere.
If I honor the elisions, I'll be fine.
I'm the blank on every document I sign.

Jana Harris

CUTTING HER OUT FROM THE FLOCK

Wagonwheel George, Cold Creek, Montana 1888

Always handle ladies the same
as livestock. When a team of fillies
bedecked in the latest boulevard fashions
stampedes the plank walkways of Billings;
air your chamber pot out of sight, then
saunter 'round to the hitch-racks lining Main.
Remember how Shep works the ewes then
cuts one from the flock? Don't let
the gals bunch together,
keep 'em moving and don't scare
your lamb by barking.
Don't rush her, let her have
her way unless she breaks
for freedom. Like buying a horse
give your lady the once over:
Born to a range mare, but carries
her head like a Hambiltonian?
Hide sleek, hair chestnut, body slender,
legs (what you can see of them) long?
If you take her dancing, all the better
to inspect her fetlocks, eyes, nose and
especially her teeth—a full string
of pearls, none long or yellow or missing.

Crazy as a barb pony?
Harder to rope than a bumblebee?
You're not looking for flashy
or fool's gold, but a soul like Old Baldy,
the lead cow you'd never sell.
Sure she might pull a pout, but
like your best roping horse, your future wife
needs to be a steady plugger.
Does she wheeze?

Of the temperament to take
a hunk of your hide? Skittish and snorting
with dissatisfaction? As to her eyes,
there comes the question: dark or light?
Remember Shep's marbled blues?
Hair color? Like herd dogs, ebonies
prove the hardest workers.
When estimating female character,
the wilder the more faithful—
the harder to break the more desirable;
a gal who'll give you her last ounce
of strength. Forget the locoed,
the jumpy or unusually dumb, probably headed
for a bender of running into buttes
or over cliffs. A locoed women's
sweet song soon turns
to something between the harangue
of a blue-tail fly and a diamondback's rattle.
If you don't want dreams filled with serpents,
give the locoed wide wagon room.

The sum essence of it all:
so she's not long on looks or faster
than her sister; she's dependable,
chunky but wise, clumsy but turns
on a silver dollar—coolheaded and sure-footed
is what'll save you. She'll jog trot when
a blizzard strikes, facing into it
all the way home; your feet
so numb you have to dismount, cling
to her mane, clutch at her bridle
following afoot in order to keep warm.
She'll never miss a step, steady up steep hills,
around cutbacks where if she slipped you'd
fall to an icy death. Even if you can't see

to steer nothing rattles her not even
the small mite of bad language needed
to encourage her on.

So suppose you cut her from the herd,
get engaged in record time, but
discover there's some meanness
in her hide or a poor water supply on her ranch
or her kin's a red-eyed coterie of rascals.
Using the excuse of your daily obscenity,
head out back to the necessary house,
lock yourself in with a bottle
of refreshment strong enough to cure
the snake bite of melancholia,
take a swig and heave
a long slow sigh more of relief
than sorrow.

Jana Harris

ABOUT THESE TRUMPETERS THAT LINE MY WALLS

Elizabeth Shepard Holtgrieve, b. 1840

Mother died in Iowa
the Christmas I was nine;
just before we went west.
Ten years after meeting Father,
my stepmother died. They first
saw each other near a Boise River switchback
when our wagon train joined hers.
Two days later, Father told Miss Nelson
they ought to take advantage
of a preacher being present
and get married. I remember
Miss Nelson bringing her things to our wagon,
we'd not much room to begin with.
I slept outside under the running gear,
awakening to . . . white foals swimming
in the backwater? No—
swans, the first I'd ever seen.
Just before Father's wedding, a little playmate
took fever and died. Another thing
I'm not likely to forget about that terrible
cholera summer of '52: a few miles east
of The Dalles we passed a wagon pulled
to the side of the road: Seven children
cowering inside. Their parents had died
and they didn't know what to do.
I'll always remember the polish in the little boy's
frightened nut-brown eyes. I tried to comfort him:
surely swans had taken his parents to heaven
along with my friend. When I got to know
Miss Nelson, I wanted to be like her.
Once, after we'd settled here on Columbia Slough,
Father cursed up a cyclone because

our boat commenced sinking and nobody'd
thought to bring a dipper. My stepmother
bailed water with her sunbonnet which saved us.

That little boy's eyes sweated
through my thoughts as I cut brush
clearing father's land.
Rafting to Portland to buy fruit trees,
we spent the night in the hut
of a boatman who had a friend in want
of a wife, a situation which pulled
up the tips of Father's down turned
horseshoe-shaped mouth.
To my amazement, Father arranged it
so that this friend would come up river to our place
in two weeks—his 28th birthday—
and we'd marry. I was 14.
Henry and I did our courting during the three
days it took to paddle to his claim.

At times the small lake on our place
blackened with ducks and geese.
Next minute I'd look up
from a colicky baby or doctoring a cow,
the pond a frothy white—great flocks
of wintering swans touched down here;
you can't imagine the noise. It even
affected the herd, their udders
tightened, we'd less milk to sell. Birds
the size of bateaux, vast wings flapping
like mainsails. Their bugling
caused so many unspeakable visions to fly
unbidden into my head—I thought
the Rapture'd come.

Now, other than the likenesses
of white trumpeters framed on my walls,
I haven't seen a swan in years.
My daughters Oceana and Henrietta
married and moved away, Charlie
lives with me, Mary is dead, John farms
the old place. You would have heard
of Arianne—her drawings of swans here
look just like life—but she died young;
Ben farms our place out on the slough;
my eldest, Emma (some mistook us
for sisters), married Zachariah Fitzgerald—
you remember him, the boy
in the wagon on the side of the road
whose parents had died, the one with polish
in his nut brown eyes.

Garrett Hongo

ON THE ORIGIN OF BLIND-BOY LILIKOI

I came out of Hilo, on the island of Hawaiʻi,
lap-steel and dobro like outriggers on either side of me,
shamisen strapped to my back as I went up the gangplank
to the City of Tokio running inter-island
to Honolulu and the big, pink hotel on Waikīkī
where all the work was back in those days.
I bought a white linen suit on Hotel Street
as soon as I landed, bought a white Panama too,
and put the Jack of Diamonds in my hatband for luck.
Of my own, I had only one song, "Hilo March,"
and I played it everywhere, to anyone who would listen,
walking all the way from the Aloha Tower to Waikīkī,
wearing out my old sandals along the way.
But that's okay. I got to the Banyan Tree
on Kalakaua and played for the tourists there.
The bartenders didn't kick me out or ask for much back.
Zatoh-no-bozu, nah! I went put on the dark glasses and pretend I
   blind.
I played the slack-key, some hulas, an island rag,
and made the tourists laugh singing *hapa*-haole songs,
half English, half Hawaiian. Come sundown, though,
I had to shoo—the contract entertainers would be along,
and they didn't want *manini* like me
stealing the tips, cockroach the attention.
I'd ride the trolley back to Hotel Street
and Chinatown then, change in my pocket,
find a dive on Mauna Kea and play *chang-a-lang*
with the Portagee, *paniolo* music with Hawaiians,
slack-key with anybody, singing harmonies,
waiting for my chance to bring out the *shamisen.*
But there hardly ever was. Japanee people
no come the bars and brothels like before.

After a while, I give up and just play whatever,
dueling with ukulele players for fun,
trading licks, make ass, practicing that
happy-go-lucky all the tourists seem to love.
But smiling no good for me. I like the stone-face,
the no-emotion-go-show on the face,
all feeling in my singing and playing instead.
That's why Japanee style suits me best.
Shigin and *gunka*, ballads about warriors
and soldier song in Japanee speech.
I like the key. I like the slap and barong of *shamisen*.
It make me feel like I galvanize
and the rain go drum on me,
make the steel go ring inside.
Ass when I feel, you know, ass when I right.
Ass why me, I like the blues. Hear 'em first time
from one *kurombo* seaman from New Orleans.
He come off his ship from Hilo Bay, walking downtown
in front the S. Hata General Store
on his way to Manono Street looking for
one crap game or play cards or something.
I sitting barber shop, doing nutting but reading book.
He singing, yeah? sounding good but sad.
And den he bring his funny guitar from case,
all steel and silver with plenty *puka* holes all over the box.
Make the tin-kine sound, good for vibrate.
Make dakine shake innah bones sound,
like one engine innah blood. Penetrate.
He teach me all kine songs. Field hollers, he say,
dakine slave g'on use for call each oddah
from field to field. Ju'like cane workers.
And rags and marches and blues all make up

from diss black buggah from Yazoo City,
up-river and a ways, the blues man say.
Spooky. No can forget. Ass how I learn for sing.

> Farewell to my baby,
> Farewell to my love.
> The guards they taking me,
> One convict in the rain.
> I going far across the sea, you know,
> And I no go'n' be home again.

Christopher Howell

MEANING

Larry should be at the meeting with Brian.
Cathy and Nancy need to know this, too,
otherwise we might have some explaining to do
with Phil! And you know how he gets.
Last time, I remember, when Eva did that thing
to the butter during lunch, Phil told Shyla
to tell Ludo to tell Eva she needed to clean
up her act because what kind of schmuck
did she think he was going to put up with
anyway, and you could tell he meant it
even though I wasn't there, actually, I heard it
later from Carol. And you heard about her and Don?
No? Well, you're the only one then. Honestly!
Those two! Well, what can you do? I mean
you have to know your cleaning products,
otherwise, you might make the same mistake,
just not where anyone could see the stripes
is all. Then, of course, there's Susan: she does it
all the time! I wonder how you bend over
like that. Next time I'll ask Lloyd to take better notes,
though it's hard to write with all that going on
and Michael right in the next room
and the cows and all. Well, back to work, I guess.
Did you want some more of this? Really?
Because if you do I can sure give it to you.

Christopher Howell

FIRST TOUCH

After the movie, the garden golf,
coffee, and long soulful walk,
after the alternating daisy petals
of elation dejection elation, we stood
in the klieg lights on her front porch.
I could hear through the door
the ox-like breathing of her father
poised to fling it wide and pounce.
From the roundness of her green eyes
I could tell she heard it too.

But inside us some kind of execution
was on the way, and we were its last meal,
our mouths beginning to know this
and to open, slightly and drift toward each other
like clouds.

We had been kissing for months.
This kiss was not that
country, this one
had nothing to do with gratitude
or the sort of evening we had had
or expectation
or revenge against nosey parents and the church
or even curiosity.
It was the exclusivity of desire,
the dizzy mutually sudden focus of our young neurons
driving us onto a single unrepeatable moment
of physical revelation fused to a steam
of lips and tongues and interpenetrating breath.

When at last we disengaged from that
eternity, still
holding me, she turned her back to the door, took
my hand and, in a gesture ceremonially exact, placed it
upon her breast.

She was wearing a bra (presumably), a blouse, a sweater
and a coat. She might have been Joan of Arc
arrayed for battle.
Nevertheless, the magnitude of this gift
surged up my arm, neck, and into my hair
till I began to lift
or faint
and felt the moon raking my blood with gems.

She drew away, smiled a little, and opened the door.
Her father, standing like Stonehenge
against the living room light, allowed her in
then shut the whole house, hard, the lion-headed
brass knocker banging like a gunshot.

I moved throbbingly down the steps and headed home.
After a block or so I could walk
normally. The softness of her lips and tongue,
that roundness and tension beneath my palm
as she held it to her, every step
brought these and such a warm loneliness
came over me, I thought I would not much mind death
then, if gods *could* die.

I walked down Hawthorn Street from 82nd to 89th
through a hall of overhanging trees, through the small
kivas of light that fell from the streetlamps.
Did I continue on Hawthorn to 92nd or turn left and cross the
    dark school yard?
It was a long time ago. Kennedy was President; Viet Nam
just a place we sent "Advisors."
Moths were circling the porch lights and dying
in ecstasies of brilliance
No one in the world but her
knew where I was.

Christopher Howell

THE NEW ORPHEUS

—*for Emma (1981–2001)*

As though windows had been nailed shut
I look out at the blank insides
of my eyes. Who lives here
in fire so deep it loves the water?
A handful of shells and a peacock moon
lie down in the dark of my arm.
Pins and needles, sorrow and salt: I'm trying
hard to match things up
with their Platonic other shinings.
I need more time for this
place I need to open like a door of rain,
like everything coming down
because of blue saturations of the unforgettable
and too hard to know. I'm giving myself just one
more lifetime of prying and pulling
at my hinges, beating the old empty roses
my daughter walks in, thinking I've been away
too long now, it's getting late, they're slamming
the other world and dousing the lights.
Rain and rain again, old winter. It's really dark
where she is. All night I lie awake
building a ladder of light.

Henry Hughes

STEELHEAD ALMOST

Too dark to retie,
they walk fishless over the bridge,
break-down rods and unboot
for the dry drive home.
Oh well, one man says. *That's fishing.*
The other doesn't want to talk. There's a barbecue tomorrow.
If you catch something, she said. *That'd be wonderful.*

Following headlights, he feels again
                    that strike behind the stone—
            cherry-blushed chrome, leapsilver and dive.
Then gone. Canyon pouring river,
swallows spading air. The trees shrug
as if nothing happened.

In a hole deeper than sleep,
    the steelhead
                    undulates fragrance and flow,
                        nudging forward—
three thousand orangey eggs
in her bright sleeve.

Henry Hughes

GUARDING THE DUMP

Karen's credit cards, Dick's drinking,
the mechanic who asked-out Mom
and left her tailpipe hanging.
It's understood. I just listen. Pile it between my ears.
Now there's my little pregnant pothead niece,
and her wacko boyfriend shooting crows
behind the dumpsters. The .22 pops.
Pops. A civil period
behind each report.

In medieval times
they guarded dumps. A busted soldier, a handsome
arrowshocked mute who liked the cry of gulls
and crazy cats, diamond flies buzzing
his fisted vaults. He'd know the rewards of silence
when the king's wagons dropped their bones,
when the surgeon's willowy wife
skirted down with her greasy basket of smiles.

Henry Hughes

TOGETHER IN THE ICE-STORM

I'd pour burning vodka over the trees
if it would help
melt that killing weight. The thought works
for a while, until sadness extinguishes
anger's blue flames
and your hair drops long
into the white basin.
I'm sorry, I say, touching your back.
But you can't hear below those creamy falls,
roots slipping from tunnels of autumn's love
before the right breast sunk, before the chemo
and the Pacific sky
surprising with combination trouble—
a little harmless snow, then freezing rain, then cold cold.
Even the evolved go down like dinosaurs
in an ice-storm.

Smoking a cigarette on the porch,
I hear the gunshot crack of a limb
that might save a groaning maple.
If only we'd make it to the sun—
crystal pains letting go
and shattering to earth
like windows of a cruel church.
Back inside for another drink, I see clippers
and a towel. I see your bald crown in firelight.
You're beautiful, I say, so close to truth
it catches and burns.

Lawson Fusao Inada

From THE WINTER OF BRIDGES

I.
That was the winter of bridges.
And, within that lofty span,
I managed to fall from one.

Oh, it wasn't much of a drop—
just a wide-mouthed plunge
about my childhood height—

and though I righted myself,
I had help up the embankment.

II.
And it was barely a bridge—
just some precarious planks
about the length of parents—

a simple short-cut among more
complex obstacles and hazards.

IV.
Not that we were adventuring—
just repeating the rounds
of rectangular confinement:

communal latrine, mess hall,
communal rock/paper/scissors . . .

It was war; get used to it.

VII.
Meanwhile, in the suspension
of furlough, a visiting uncle
had issued me his overcoat:

"a robin's-egg blue," imbued
with auras of campus dances,
jazzy trips over the bridge
to illustrious San Francisco.

Major alteration was planned.
Handiwork for a hand-me-down
by barrack light, a mother
meticulously materializing,
conforming California to fit.

IX.
. . . I took the trench, the spatter;
I took the drench, the shudder:
I took the stench, the sputter;

I took whatever I contracted—

the spiraling fevers, delirium—

but: I will not take it again.

X.
As for that coat, no matter.

It served its tour of duty
in a camouflaged condition

only to become one casualty
of our subsequent captivity

in Colorado, where an uncle,
from his outfit in Wyoming,

provided a fitting garment:

A cowboy jacket. American.

XIII.
There—that can last a while.
Minor alteration as planned.

Reinforcement for stability
Nothing to look at or notice.

A decked-out, cautionary kid
can cross without incident.

Elders will not be standing
vigil by a convulsing child.

XV.
Vigil on a bolstered bridge.
Searchlights through storm.

In the name of the war effort—
to slap this squalor together.

In the name of the war effort—
to slip currency into coffers.

Bulldozers, bonfires, mounds:
The defilement jutting rubble . . .

Laura Jensen

BIRD THAT FELL TO THE GROUND

In the falling and rising
Of its breast remember
Trying to run through water
And that dream. It lay
On frozen wings
Large in shock and need.
Up. Down. And the fallen
Made its fast sound,
Sprang from the shadow
To a branch in the sun.

What came between
Is old and young.
"What can I do?"
I asked a woodpecker.
Knowledge of hands
And knowledge of tongue,
One incongruous, one one.

Laura Jensen

FOUR SUMMER OUTFITS

Pigeons, railroad tracks
and butterfly bushes,
one wing anima, one animus.
Also those stuck skin legs
on a bus seat in hot weather
Meditate on a fascination
with the other.
Any structure or idea
rock walls
when the law of metal owns.

Like a chain link fence
along a trail. Past the fresh links
the crumbles of dust
half bury dim log steps.

Days, weeks, I emailed
Representative Darneille.
Librarians showed me internet
in 1999 and I am fifty-four.
When I click sometimes I go outside,
where they are.
I hallucinate her across the white
hard street in summer purple.
I do not step into the street.
She speaks on the other side.

They did it about six months ago.
The City. There were homeless camps.
But they just go around the end.

There are Canada Geese
and the billowing smoke
far along to the south
is the color of them.

The information overload
is a warehouse burning
that was a hundred and two years old.
It stayed forever in my periphery.
And it seems a tumbling domino
that the conflagration
can have small effect

on a Sunday head count
at old Lutherische, which is
across the street from it
like a carved toy
it dropped when it stumbled
and started crying.

They showed me word processor
in 2000. We know Lutherische
has a red line under it,
that I have an emotional cloud
all around me. Once
on a bus that was a pity.
But Lutherische has a red line
under it, again.

A woman's black long clothes
climb the gray clouds into the sky
instead of standing still as she walks
in the photo on the street in the city.

But my poem is like getting a tan.
We want it deep and deep.
Like a model lies on a beach
in the magazine. And there is a story
about a restored building.

And the magazine is on sale
at a supermarket, and
there we cannot remember
that it is too bad about the building.
We wear the same
t-shirts in the summer weather.
No one is someone I know,
even when something is wrong
like this. All strangers.

Laura Jensen

FLAGS—JANUARY 1999

On the wide lawn little flags at the holes.
From beneath shade trees and evergreen
along the driveway
these little flags were not noticeable.
In the sunlight—

For so long I have walked
very easily and hardly want to sit down.

Suppose the garter snake rolled down
to the surface of the pond like a mirror.
Suppose the sailboat looked too—
into the still water at its reflection
and how sun prising it had been so long.

The very small figure balanced on
the very small surfboard in the wave of ocean
the bee all loaded with pollen
flies right by him, it is balanced on
something else, and at the tip of its stinger
is a tiny barb—

It swings away in a circle on a wing.
And all of these beauties of the light
are about my mother—how many times
all the planes of color
have been about absence even when
the air was so clear I did not remember.

But the grief that was there, it left
small scratches on us everywhere.

Laura Jensen

ROBINS IN THE DARK

Three dark birds on the sidewalk, the parking
where the grass that would be ice
but is not haloes in the streetlamps.
In the lamps on the houses and small lawns,
backlit sillouettes.

Then a dull sound,
a flat gong on the cement lamppost ahead,
one with a wheeled cart and a white crutch
crosses on the walk sign.

The far distance straight ahead is two health
and hospital monoliths.
Across the street a solid modern church,
the cement cross in the courtyard
shapes upward smaller to seem
it is flying off into the sky.

At the near hospital months ago
a woman shot herself
and the one with the wheeled cart
steps up beside the smell of the fire
that burned the El Toro—the Bavarian—
the smell of the booths and the coffee machine,
the wooden carved woodwork all pulled out,
a few burnt china soup cups and a yellow
CAUTION band. No one was hurt.

The places of violence reclaimed
by the Allied Ministries now
refers the far distance to the aspiration
and the beauty of the presbyterian
congregation.
When day begins a shrub beside
the old building fills with sounds of birds.

Jonathan Johnson

THREE CAFÉS

Someone, Pietro, somewhere, in Italy,
with his own sense of leisure, Pinot Noir,
and articulation, sketchbook, sits outside at a café
he thinks of as his, that spot in creation
where wind sends its cool breeze
across his loose shirt without riffling his pages.

He thinks no other light gives like this light and
of course he's right.
                        As is Antonio
who sees it as lonely, in another district
of the same small city, at his own café,
getting right the widow's monologue
in his new play while pigeons watch
and the fountain gurgles away. Pietro and Antonio
have never met, though they'd recognize
each other, being of an age, late twenties,
and both spending so much time alone in public
the last couple years—the cinema, walking
the road lined with Lombardy poplars
beside the bay, the market every Saturday.

Pietro buys bananas; Antonio bread.
Pietro rents a room; Antonio's father is dead.

He lives at home with his mother
and seventeen-year-old sister, Nicoletta, with whom
he's worked to stay close. Evenings,
at the kitchen table, they often play chess.
Their mother does the dinner dishes.
Their father had a policy, so Antonio
needn't work. He should write, his mother insists,
and stay home for Nico (though soon she'll
be off to Parma for University).

Pietro tacks his sketches, the few he likes,
to the wall in his room. His favorite
is of two girls on bikes. The first girl
glances over her shoulder at the other
behind her, that sunny wind he knows so well
in her hair.
      And meanwhile here, at my café,
countries, an ocean, and states away, I imagine
her riding past him, and in my own
sun and leisure and new love of Pietro and Antonio
consider whether she should be Nico
or some other girl, someone none of us knows.

Jonathan Johnson

SURPLUS

I don't want to be here
   to think of all the sex
in the six-foot stack
   of spent dorm mattresses,
a dollar a piece,

or the years of eyes
   that strained for some glimmer
of understanding just beyond
   these computer screens, as blank
in rows on folding tables

as night after night
   of overcast above
the observatory, where
   someone waited to show
what he knew of eternity.

There's too much importance,
   too much of you and me
out among the sunlit benches,
   library steps and hedges
of today to stay

sifting racks of warm-up pants
   for a pair my size
and running my fingers
   over the coffee circle stained
veneer of someone's desk

who also spent some days
   at the sunlit pinnacle
of history, doing
   serious work, no doubt,
wholly in the moment

once in a while—
   the smell of coffee,
solidity of this desk
   and beautiful thoughts
no one's bothered to salvage.

Arlitia Jones

A WINTER FAIRYTALE

The moon is just
the moon and not a white doe
standing still in a forest of stars
and that is simply a dog

barking off in the night
and not the ancient wolf
baying, crouched, waiting to leap
and pull the moon down

and gore it on top of new snow
which is never a silvered robe
of silk draped over the earth.
The snow is simply snow.

Why do poets make this mistake?
We insist on so much more,
it's not enough the moon is the moon,
full, celestial and distant.

Would no one believe us if we said
the dog is brown, mongrel and thirsty?
The man who owns him
did not feed him today,

why should he change his old habit?
The dog is scared, chained to a truck.
He makes a weird dance
lifting each paw in turn

because his smooth pads
sting when they touch the ice.
Ah, night, clear and arctic and long.
Is this not credible?

Poets, quit thumbing your book of myths.
Don't speak to us of the grandiose music
of heaven or lead us with the velvet shoulder
of darkness that carries us forward to dawn.

Look and see the light that comes on
in the window of the house
farther down the moonspit valley
where an angry wife who is not

a good witch, hands a rifle
to her husband who is a huntsman
because she has to open up the shop
in the morning, because she's desparate

for a few hours sleep, and she's had it
with the damn dog, with the night's injustice.
Write what she said.
Please, do this for me.

Eve Joseph

OLD AGE

It surprises me each time
I see a horse lie down in a field

a protest

in the bend and fold:
the way a body relinquishes its hold
as it sinks, unguarded,
to the earth.

Eve Joseph

AVALANCHE

A white mountain
shifts in the mind—
above treeline
four men

begin their ascent,
a dragon's cry
the groan of ice
and they are boys again—

armed with sword and scabbard,
pearl-handled guns;
what do they know

of fracture? A step, forward.
Winter apples. Winter sun.
A cornice and the thin blue nothing below.

Richard Kenney

SURREALISM

Skillet bottom rule-straight prairie releasing a little
To a ripple of sand hills, side-lit

At twilight, called The Palouse. Note again schooling fishes
Nosing the windscreen, uffish

Through the sunroof. Whites pooled at the bottoms of my eyes,
I watch a spiky caudal fin surmise,

Ripple, and disappear. *I hate surrealism,*
You say, sullen. *How do you feel about nonsense, lissome*

One, I rejoin, adding *ghogli woolly scrooly lo.*
Och, wholly different, family and phylum! you yell, O

You prefer History . . . deep History,
The *really* used to, the *true,* the *facts,* austere,

Where the sand hills of the Palouse surippidly rumple on
Like the pink roof of the doggish yawn,

Formed as they were in the outrushing tidal estuary
Of the Mid-Cretaceous Seaway, where

We speak, right here, and above,
To a depth of a hundred feet at least, my scurrily love.

Richard Kenney

REAR VIEW

At 90 on I-90 out of Anaconda,
Montana, a lone deinonychid biker— look,
He's passing: he's taking the road like a dog on a leg,
Or the flatulent jump of a Thompson gun . . .

Condor neck, gray mane a coronal storm
Around his plastic yarmulke— the logos
That pate sports relate mostly to the holocaust
Between his legs, the verbs for which he's said "to be born."

His own shanks canted high as a birthing mother's
Leave him in semi-reclining elegance.
Claws clung up wide high like Christ's. Fringed leggings,
Jerkin, gauntlets, thongs—he's clothèd all in leather.

I watch his flogging shadow, thrown noon-low
Below the chassis. It writhes like a count's cape
Caught in a belt sander: so the paved
Miles howl by, and who'll alone

As on a Harley or a desert island not gape
A little in the rear-view mirror? Meanwhile, the fringe
On his saddlebags whips nicely. Inside . . . a syringe?
A Glock or two? Ibuprofen? Books On Tape?

A flick of the wrist, a puff of blue, and this god's
Gone. Thoughts of the road. Long thoughts.

Richard Kenney

PATHETIC FALLACY

The rocks look wrinkled
and the sea, sore

and what do the willows
know of war?

The king in his orchid
curdles noon

till the stars are salt
in the western wound.

And when and when
the baby cries

the moon leaks milk
in the rooster skies,

and so and so
till morn is eve

once more as ever
but make believe.

Richard Kenney

SHALL I COMPARE THEE TO APPEARANCES?

I check my watch. 8:10. You paint an eye, blinking
In the dubious glass held up to the Christmas party,
Turning back the clock. You are very pretty,
But also beautiful; but what I'm thinking

Is: Rainier. Invisible all month behind a veiling
Weather one wouldn't have thought could cloak a moth-
Wing, well, tonight the ancient volcano, big as the mother
Of all mother ships, shows its alien

Glacier to the moon. It looks close enough to lick.
And how much worse than a lamp-post, that. And all along,
Who cared a fig for anything but the long
And short and heavy and high and wide? Here's to the relic

Of the what else, wet on the nerve, and what compares?
Numbers?

Richard Kenney

TURBULENCE

> *On his death bed, Werner Heisenberg declared that he will have two*
> *questions for God: "why relativity, and why turbulence." Heisenberg*
> *said, "I really think He may have an answer to the first question."*

There is of course the nervous question of the airfoil;
Laminar flow through the headphones where wave-torque
Puddles the brains of my seatmate; awful

Rockaddle; also, missing shards of crockery tucked
Behind our unplugged refrigerator, as bits
Of Mars are littering Antarctica.

Consider, too, the impudence of fluids,
How when my double gurgles off the little iceberg
Of its highball, one drop often finds the eye. Follow it

Where the penny, bouncing from the urban cobble, spark
In a pocket, arcs elsewhere, and winds up spinning
From the Bridge of Sighs. Let's say God's spigot

Needs a washer, which you, while explaining
Physics to a friend, supply. Chaos,
is all, you yawn, sleepily—not in the splenetic

Literary-critical sense, requiring Icarus
To fall and fall and fall, but rather in the rinsing,
Sundog, water-scatter sense, here in the cirrus

Of it all, that pure ebulliance we're (as
The bubbly flight attendant says) experiencing.

Michael Kenyon

FEAST

> *Now come, the last that I can recognize,*
> *pain, utter pain, fierce in the body's texture.*
> *As once in the mind I burned, so now I burn*
> *in you; the wood resisted, long denied*
>   *—Rilke*

A child in winter under the sickle
moon one moment is bright with play, in love
with candy, lips and fingers Smartie red
(she likes red best), cartwheels on black branches,
oak branches written by wind and street lamp
on the hardwood floor, next moment's surprised
by a cloud that mixes moon with sweetness,
cartwheel with voices from the kitchen, Mom
and Auntie, who discuss olives and lies.
Now come, the last that I can recognize,

old mountain beacon that holds fast sun's light,
though all agree it's nearly night, and bring
news of wealth, gold, the latest adventures
of gods adrift far from the shore, no wind,
oarless, trying to get home by dreams of
red cows full of milk in such green pasture
foccacia, arugula, lettuce,
balsamic vinegar and oil, white plates,
rectory table, subtract from pleasure
pain, utter pain, fierce in the body's texture.

That moon, that child, divide heaven's promise
between them; the good food turns grey when day's
hue is absorbed, and streets, hedges, palings,
all turn grey. Then mortal families gather,
women's lies no stronger than lies of men,
too flushed to sit down, while the children learn
there's slippage, a hole in the sky, the skin,
some wrong thing among them that burns and burns
the way wine, dark red, dries the throat and burns.
As once in the mind I burned, so now I burn

to heal this hurt child, light new white candles,
start the feast. She tells us she feels sick, can't
stand the noise. All lies cease, laughter bows out.
A child sickens in January. Spring
breaches. A branch taps the window. She runs
in circles. With no one sober we hide
our fear and call a cab. Again the rush
of sudden fog: I'm in my first forest,
mouth zeroed. O trees, we want to confide
in you; the wood resisted, long denied

Joanna Klink

WHAT (WAR 2003–)

And if all those who meet or even
hear of you become witness to what you are—
a white country of blight beneath the last

snows of spring. Could we remain quiet on earth
and bear it, the war we make inside what is,
a sound dense with sleep and chemicals,

the raw space between words. It's a long time
to be here, to be still, to feel the rot inside
now—bone-dust, char, sheets of stars

at the edge of a field where we are once again
taken from ourselves. Could we remain here,
witness to grief, one last bright dire call-and-

reply, each bird-cry or siren extinguished
where some trueness abides, some portion
we have lost our right to claim or know.

It comes into any mind that would perceive it,
leaf-rot, speech-rot, the deliberate ribcage of the deer,
these abrupt chalk cliffs over which

the confused animals fling themselves, and you, obscure,
receive no response that is not suffered
as the days grow long and distortions

come to seem the natural course of things—
what badly snapped tree-limbs whose creatures
stray into space—and they find they cannot land

though the stark white eyelid struggles
open—no answer, no resolution—
a window opened to the mute green world,

weedy and driftless, a wind drilling rain, dirt,
the parameters of uncertainty, of hope,
what we might be against what we have done,

bees crawling in the mouth of the one
who would say *the earth turned into sour flesh,*
the sweetness into horror—what strange rooms,

what soundless movement of sky over desert
where the flesh again is beaten and the emptiness
extends itself while some old man looks on,

an entry in a book, the sand-field around him
blown thinly toward sun, or the moths
clustered against unnatural embers, no longer

ourselves in the afternoons, evenings,
weak, vague, clutched at the mouth—
because we did nothing, because we lost count.

Joanna Klink

OPEN LAND

When would I be willing to hide nothing,
as in mid-autumn the fields are cleared and turned
without great struggle or abandon, the dark blue

storms arriving in patterns of lush thunder,
a cool spray spun back from the grass.
As if the smaller, truer meanings could be partially

deciphered (a birch just a piece of what was once
a star, the stars behind the clouds in silver, living
tissue). Yet here it is: a tree turned

white by rain, its roots immobile, and next to it,
fields of indistinguishable crop that seem
composed, or blank, or unwilling to be made clear.

*

And you, how you stayed here anyway,
close to that baffling interior, the light-gray
milky air at the edge of the lake, holding out

some constant promise of understanding.
Explain then how it could continue, this steady
privacy, this ice, iridescent and hard liquid,

the water caught in merciful, unwavering
shades of white. Winters passed. The lines
were cut deeply by skaters, violet as the laws

of size, shape, and brightness required.
I moved the words in my head,
trying to say what it has meant.

One either sleeps or wakens. One begins
again, in graying sunshine, last night's rain
damp silver on the grass. And the world

does nothing to make the way more clear,
and my voice, which would say simply what is there—
the creek-chords of rushing water,

the boarded houses scrubbed with salt—
trips on the minor, stinging details (this fence—
how can its shadow go so long unchanged?).

How to love you freely, with uncompromising
honesty, as a birch might pass through fog
and stay the same, this same tree,

though the black weather persist and days
already lived accept no true correction.
Is there time—will you listen—do I have

speech enough? What words do is
everything. The sky clouds and then breaks open—
a sweetness scattered over these dark trees.

Joanna Klink

EXCERPTS FROM A SECRET PROPHECY

You who never turned from me,
who were near from the start.
And when I found no prospect of change,
even in the workings of sunshine, you pulled
the coat around me and said nothing.
And the river moved, a slow crush of ice
through the dark dawn. And it wasn't confusion,
and it wasn't grief in the wind, but something
disordered, an isolation over many seasons,
the presence and withdrawal of light on the sealine,
incongruencies of shells. And everywhere
arising and perishing, the tidal life driven by pattern,
division, imbricate distances of dusk across the lawn,
deep summer, a weight in the air
blurring soft against our eyes—this world, these backyards,
the air loose with birds, a dream
that comes from below as the heart pumps
blood on the steady threshold of emptiness.
Aubade of the northern country where every ocean
is imagined, aubade of light falling across
the vast migrations, a hint of extinction in each wing,

aubade of the old fairgrounds, the vacant orchards
shifting soundlessly in snow—an inwardness
that belongs to the stars and tides, flickering in circuit
between your breath and the clouds, aubade of clouds,
of reperception and sorrow, dark eyes, inconstancy,
everything I have tried to explain, sparse aubade
of the weekend minutes, wild mint, evenings
when we hear the scrape of moths at screenlight,
and always barn swallows banking in the jewel periphery,
always our skin gathering age, in time to be emptied,
in time scarcely recognized—

Why did we live?
                 Apparitions beneath
the slow turning of stars, distilled in bodies
that bruise even when walking softly, unsafe,
unanswered within a world that does not close,
but opens, constantly opens, rain and snow on the river,
these reeds breaking through sheets of ice toward sun—
and the language you choose, and what you have chosen
to say to me each day, your voice returning me
to shadow, snowdrift, the constant messages of air,
sweeping pattern within each breath-note—
wren, bed, person, circumstance—
yours and mine, yours, you
who are so at home in words,
who were lost from the start.

Patrick Lane

THE WAR

Afternoon, and the heat upon the table slipped across the
    melmac plates
and the steel knives and the butter, melted from the plastic
    saucer, slipped
to the edge of the scarred pine table and sank to the linoleum.
    Heat
like the pale water you see on desert roads ahead of you, the
    shimmer
and the mirage of a lake reflected from the bellies of clouds,
    you drive
through thirsty, the wheel wet under your palms. Before us
    water glasses
beaded from the sweat of air when the cold meets it, the home-
    made beer
thin with foam. He lived above Swan Lake and made pottery
    there,
celadon and slip glazes drawn from the yellow clay cliffs,
    temmoku,
the rabbit's-fur black running down, feldspar, iron, copper, and
    the ashes
from bones, calcium and phosphorous, ball clays and kaolin, all
for his huge hands to make into the empty containers others
    filled
with flowers, the vitrified glass, what he was proud of, a frail
    red rising
out of a deeper brown, the black, the impurities, the polluting
    elements,
and the beauty of his making. He was a German, come over
    after the war,
and the same age as me, his parents dead, I think, or if not dead
then never spoken of. His hand reached through the air for
    bread,
broke off the crust at the end, and then he ate it, slowly,
    between

sips of beer. We talked the way men talked back then when they spoke
of the past, a privacy only spoken to wives and rarely then, the older days
best kept where they were in the locked leather satchel of the heart.

His was a long story that came slowly out of silence
and told without his eyes looking at me, but staring instead
out the window at the stubborn apples ripening, a pale brush of fire
flaring under the hard green. Summer in the Okanagan. The heat
and a single fly and then sweeping slowly, catching the fly as it rose
backwards as flies do when they first lift from what they rest on, bread,
the crumbs fallen on the slick surface of the table, a lick of wet butter.
He held his fist to my ear so I could hear the buzzing
then flung the fly to the floor, the single sharp click of its body
breaking there. And the story going on, the fly an interruption
he seemed unaware of except for the holding it to my ear
to hear its frantic wings, its sharp death, and the bread almost gone.
I spoke of the war and how it had shaped who I was, the years
forming me, had told him of my childhood and my father
gone to fight in Europe and of my playing what we called
as children, War. How we would choose sides, the smallest kids
the enemy, the Germans, and how we would come down on them
with our wooden rifles made from broken apple boxes
and boyonet them where they lay exposed, choosing to ignore their cries
of, It's not fair. We pushed the thin blades of our rifles

into their soft bellies, their shouts and cries meaning nothing to
us
and then their tears, shameless, little kids broken in the shallow
trenches
we had made in the clay hills, imagining what our fathers did
each day
in the sure glory they never spoke of afterward, no matter our
begging.

And his story.

That he watched his father and uncle come home to their farm
in the Black Forest, the horses pulling the short wagon in the
night,
nostrils breathing mist in the cold, the wagon back piled with
straw.
and the bodies of children under the straw.
That they had hunted them down in the forest, children
run from the gathering of jews and gypsies, tattered clothes and
rags
wrapped round their feet. He remembered the small feet
hanging
from the back of the wagon, the rags like torn flags fluttering.
His father and uncle had lifted the bodies one by one and fed
them
into the grinders with dry corn and rotting turnips and
blackened potatoes,
the pigs clambering over each other and screaming.
His mother had found him watching and carried him back
into the house, swore him to silence, said what she said and
said again,
and he had not spoken of it these past thirty years and why
he spoke of it now he did not know, but that I had asked him of
the war,

and of children playing, and that he had played too, but what
  games
they were he didn't remember, it was so long ago, those years,
  that war.
But what he remembered most were the feet sticking out
from under the straw, the horses' heavy breathing, the rags
  fluttering,
and his father sitting beside his uncle, tired, staring into the
  dark barn,
and the wagon pulling heavy through the ruts,
and the rags wrapped around the feet sticking out from the
  straw,
and the rags fluttering. That. He remembered that.

In the desert hills the Ponderosa pines have grown three
  hundred years
among bluebunch wheatgrass and cheatgrass and rough fescue,
  and
there are prickly-pear cactus in spring whose flowers are made
  one each day,
and among the grasses are rabbit-brush and sagebrush and
  antelope brush
where the mountain bluebird is a startled eye, the grasshopper
  sparrow,
and the sage thrasher, and the wood mouse and harvest mouse,
and the kangaroo rats who come out at night to feed on seeds
  and moths.
There are these living things, and they are rare now and not to
  be seen
except for the careful looking in what little is left of that desert
  place. And I
list them here in a kind of breathing, the vesper sparrow, the
  saw-whet owl,
and the western meadowlark, and the northern scorpion and
  the western rattlesnake,

now almost gone, the last of them slipped away into what I
   remember
of that time when I lived among them. I name only what I can,
my friend, the potter who lived above Swan Lake, who made
   pottery
from kaoliln and ball clay and the glazes from the yellow clay
   of the hills,
and who was but a child in that far war almost no one
   remembers
now, the warrior dead, and the people dead, the men and
   women dead,
and the children dead, and the children of those warriors and
   those people
who remember are now fewer than they were, and that is how
   it is now.

Sage thrasher, wood mouse, western meadowlark, and saw-
   whet owl,
and the meadowlark, and the vesper sparrow, and rough fescue,
and I must tell you so you understand, that we sat there at that
   table
with cold glasses of beer and the remains of the bread we ate
   together
and he showed me how to cup my hand and come up slowly
behind a resting fly and then sweep my hand through the air
perhaps two inches from the table top, the fly who lifts
   backwards
when he flees, caught in my fist, and then flinging it to the floor,
   the click
of its body breaking there. And that I learned how to do that,
and it was important I knew what I was learning, though it was
only a kind of game between two me killing flies, and then
we went outside under the weight of the heavy sun and talked a
   moment,

and he did not speak of his crying at the table and I did not
    speak of it,
for we were men of that time and we had learned long ago not
    to speak
of tears and of the stories that bring them, and that in this only
    world
there are things that must be remembered, and that they be
    spoke of,
scarlet gilia, parsnip-flowered buckwheat, white-tailed
    jackrabbits,
and balsamroot, and the rare sagebrush mariposa, and all such
    things
that are almost gone, and that I can still catch a fly the way
he taught me, and that we stood there by his truck in the dust
    and the heat
and said nothing to each other, only stared out into the
    orchards
and the green apples ripening there, and then he was gone into
    the desert
and I can tell you only this of what I remember of that time.

Patrick Lane

HOWL

The wolves howl with loneliness that is only theirs.
The coyotes howl with the same wish.
The solitary loons too on the mountain lakes.
I have heard them among the hills and the far valleys.
There is no sound like theirs.
I know you cannot imagine what it is like.
I know you cannot believe anything alive can make that sound.
But you will, you will.

Dorianne Laux

THE LIGHT NEXT DOOR

Morning light on the house next door,
going from gray to ochre to blaze
then back to the color the neighbor painted it
ten years ago, a sordid mid-day yellow.
Wasps burrow in the eaves, crane flies
hover over the blown down grass.
He's a political man, gone all day
and half the night, talking clean air
and land reform. His small creased car
papered in stickers:
Save the Whales. No Nukes.
He wears the same suit every day.
From my second story window
I see the bald spot growing
on top of his head. He never brings
a sack of groceries home, never
a strange woman, only rolled up posters,
boxes of stampless letters, bag brown
accordion files. Sparrows nest
in his attic vent, gather corn shocks
from my backyard garden, twigs,
scraps of trash, fluff caught in the bushes.
Jettisoned streamers of white shit
glitter down the sides of his house.
Some nights I hear him singing
to the cat, watch him through
the curtainless laundry window
as he stuffs his blue shirts
into the machine. In summer,

all he wears is socks, stepping
soundlessly through pools of lamplight,
pacing back and forth with nothing
but a task on his face, no doubt or shame,
just his vulnerable body and something
to be done. Right now he's standing
in a spear of light, peering out
his window at the disappearing world.
How could we expect him to save us?

Dorianne Laux

CAN A FIRE BURN FOREVER?

Why such devotion after all these years, this rapt
attention when he rises from the rumpled bed
or sits on a chair half-dressed to slide on his socks?

His ankles still surprise—the dear matching knobs,
the skinny veins that run beneath such papery skin.
Something in me is determined, moved

to see him again, each day, freshly. It's beyond
my comprehension or control, my body
a satellite to his even now, in its exile,
while he's away in his big car on some errand.

I need to see him standing in the doorway, returned
safe from the market, a quart of milk in one hand,
his keys dangling from the other. Can my body

follow his from room to room forever, my eyes
awed by each limb's motion as if he's a creature
from another universe, my heart an acquisitive

percussionist as he orchestrates the dirty dishes
or arranges the cans and plastics in the blue
recycling bin? Has he become my personal religion?
Exhaling Hail Marys as he leans against the doorjamb

to the distaff music of the spheres, spikes of light
crashing through the kitchen window. My eye's
daily rapture. My body's nightly polyphonic fire.

Dorianne Laux

EASTER, 1999

A week has passed since I first veered
to miss the pumpkin stranded
on the curve of road beside
the continuation high school. Kids.
Who can guess what they had in mind.
Certainly its placement is inspired: just
above the curve, out of view
until I'm already well on top of it,
my left tire skimming the orange crust.
Each day I forget, until, at the apex
of my turn I squash it again, noting,
in my rearview, the latest damage.
Who among these gangly, saw-toothed
adolescents had the inspiration, understood
the complicated physics of angle and curve?
Who whispered, No, not there. There.
Who are these children, no longer
children— not quite grown— off-spring
of TV, spawn of rock-and-roll, heirs
to the sleepless eyes of computers
and nuclear energy. The Days of Plague.
The seedless orange. They carry our future
inside their meager bodies, skimpy
arms and thighs that glide beneath a swoon
of baggy jeans, conveyors of weekend sex
and junk food, furtive as they punch each other,
defiant as they cross the street without looking
or stop to stare down a row of backed-up cars,
furious or sullen-eyed, on the brink.
I've seen them stooped on a corner
swapping cigarettes and beer or propped

against a fence, tangled around each other,
their glossy hair slipping through
open diamonds of chainlink.
I've watched them slink across a lawn
and drop their books like bombs
on the dirt, slide their fingers
into belt loops and just stand there, glaring.
Who among them found an April pumpkin
six months past its prime, who foresaw
the sweet implication of the cambered street?
Or did one of them simply kick the thing
while the others broke into a cheer?
By next week there'll be nothing
but a smear in the middle of a street
they cross every day on the way to
becoming what they hope to be.
One is climbing a tree, another is swaying
to some inner music, her books held tight
against her swollen belly and breasts
or that one, walking toward the open
auditorium door like an old man—
somber, head down, shoulders slumped in
toward his heart— who suddenly
and without apparent motive, leaps
into the air like the child
he longs to be, grabs at the overhang
with his fingers, misses,
then steps into the dark.

Ursula K. Le Guin

A MEASURE OF DESOLATION: FEBRUARY 2005

Again and again the landwind blows,
sending back the rain
to the house of the rain.

Seeking, seeking the heron goes
longlegged from creek
to thirsty creek.

They cry and cry, the windblown crows
across the sky,
the bare clear sky.

From land to land the dry wind blows
the thin dry sand
from the house of sand.

Ursula K. Le Guin

WATCHING THE FRACTAL SET

Candidates are hacked into
small bloodless morsels and deepfried
in steroids and the weather will occur while
skyscrapers and redwoods skip about
in earnest spectacles on a nose
two seconds long at most and once again
the Jesus man the zircon bargains scores
of ballgames and the round black ears
while people laugh who are not there or dead
and if you zoom up it seems larger yet
is the same size exactly or zoom down
and it seems tee-tiny but no change in size exactly
all the same the weather Jesus steroids zircons
candidates dead children laughing and
the awful round black ears with round black ears on them
with round black ears on them: the Mouse of Mandelbrot.

Tod Marshall

DESCRIBE BOOK BLURBS TO NATIONALISM

You are necessary
You are needed, you are the new you, improved, better than the
    other you's.
You combine art and electricity, ham and rye.
You are the sharp mustard between meat and cheese.
You cling like burdock, flow like river. You are to your like we
    to wet.
You house builder you state builder you democracy builder
    extreme.
You hang sheetrock with neat seams.
You paint the scenery so it seems real.
You plumb. You deep deep deep.
You wire the stars. You roof the sky.
You intelligent, brave, brilliant, honest, you risk-taker extreme.
O risky risky you.
Your precision is clearly precise.
You move, you muse, you dazzle, you brilliant.
Brilliant, brilliant you.
You genius, you incarnation, you epiphany, Virgin Mary in
    moldy bread.
You Walt Whitman mixed with Martin Luther King.
You Dickinson, Shakespeare, Dante's lost brother.
You Rome. You Byzantium.
You Marconi, you radio, you chat room, you needed.
You flag. You necessary.
O necessary you.

Tod Marshall

DESCRIBE WILDFLOWERS TO ETHICS

The ground gives a push.
The rocks applaud,
and nearby, waterfalls like rivers of joyful tears—
that time laughing so hard at my son
toddling around the house
with an erection on which he'd hung
the friendship bracelet from the Bible People
that said "What Would Jesus Do?"
Answer that one and you might be able to see
those purples, reds, and yellows,
the subtle lavender gloss, sheeny greens and pinks,
even the over-the-top oranges,
and not be tempted to pick the explosive petals
to press into a notebook
with the desperate hope
you could one day open the pages
and say *as it was, let it be.*

Try again: you are what you do:
I reddy paintbrush purply gold and greeny green green.
I Pearly Everlasting. I fillyum trillium, birdfoot violet blueflag.
I write down these scribbles of smoke,
and we sometimes see them against the sky:
The fire is always coming. And it's coming soon.

Linda McCarriston

GOD THE SYNECDOCHE IN HIS HOLY LAND

i.m. Rachel Corrie

Around you the father gods war. This
Father. That father. The other father.

What more dangerous place could
A woman stand, upright, than on that sand, as if
She were still antiphon to that voice, the other
Mind of that power. *The very idea!*

Crush her back in to her mother!
Crush her. Consensus. War.

Linda McCarriston

PUBLIC POEM IN THE FIRST PERSON

Myself, the poet, is musing
on the spiritual. Not *religion*, opium
of the people, *spirituality*
opium of the elite. Trying
I keep trying to break my mind

so it will match my heart.
"My mind's not right" Lowell
told us, and Sexton, and Plath put her mind
we know where. Poetry, I will
stand forever outside your door

in the winter square, outside
your edifice, cathedral or prison,
and never go in again, I will
stand as Keats stood with his
paper sword by the door of his
dying mother, if as I am

I am unwelcome. My mind's not
not right. Shall I come in?

Frances McCue

THE ORPHAN'S CONSOLATION

When they say, "How lucky you are! Just so lucky!"
they mean, "It was only luck that saved you."
They mean, "We felt kind that day. Our good will is your
    fortune."

When they say, "You were lucky to be clothed,"
they mean, "We gave you clothes. How kind we were!"
They mean, "We might have saved those clothes for others."

When they say, "We sent you to school. Such luck!"
they mean, "We gave you to the school."
They mean, "An education makes you worth something. You
    owe us."

When they say, "We fed you. You're just lucky we fed you,"
they mean, "some of our food. It was ours."
They mean, "We spent our money on perishables. Lucky for
    you."

When they say, "We gave you a roof over your head,"
they mean, "You are lucky. You dwelled in our kindness."
They mean, "Our house was never yours."
You know you were taken in. And it was just luck.

Robert McDowell

LET'S SAY WHAT'S ALWAYS LEFT UNSAID

On the parent playing field we stunk it up.
We tried every diet and fitness regimen
That came down the pike, but gravity won.
If we'd had the money, we'd have gone for
Liposuction, tummy tucks, implants and facelifts.
When we weakened we compromised.
There wasn't a friend we wouldn't betray
If the personal pay-off were high enough.
We hated our regional managers
And the irritating people we hung out with
In the office, and after hours in bars
Because we had no place else to go.
We romanced others because we were bored
And they just happened to show up.
When people we knew got down on their luck,
We said all the things we were supposed to say
While thinking, *thank God it's happening to him,*
Not me, that poor, pathetic sonofabitch!
With our intimates we made fun of others in distress.
We showed up at funerals acting sad and sorry
While secretly exulting: *They're dead, not us!*
Not us.

Robert McDowell

1936. HIROKO'S PASSAGE

My mother died,
My father, too,
Before I spoke
Or walked the room
Or fought my way
To where I'd be
Across the sea.

On board my bed
Was by the cook's,
A four-foot plank
That folded out
And dangled from chains.
I'd hug the wall,
Afraid I'd fall.

I knew that I
Had traveled far
From orphanage
To dock, to star,
From empty space
   And setting sun
To this new one.

Colleen J. McElroy

BALLAD FOR THE BLUE MOON TAVERN

Saturday nights when the tavern
really rocked, the girl perched
on the slice of neon moon above

the door winked while poets
gathered, their bar stools notched
like some gunslinger's belt—

certain seats reserved for hotshots
who crowded in before the fake moon
glowed full blue against

the cobalt blue of the northern night
sky:: and just for the record, the pin-up
girl kept count of who walked in

and where they sat—Dylan Thomas
there and Carolyn and David huddled
in that corner and over there

Dick Hugo—who years later sober
claimed he couldn't understand
what folks did with all that time

on their hands—but those nights
in the Blue Moon no one mentioned
time and how Dylan's days were numbered

or how long before John Logan morose
as ever stumbled home to his houseboat
where the lake spread its tawdry skirt

welcoming any moon—those nights time
was measured on Picard's barometric light
while the Blue Moon mocked the real moon

cresting above the tips of regal pines—
and the pin-up girl nested in the arc of moon
above the door asked in the spit and hiss

of tubing which one cast the best
light and which held the most stars
in its sway:: on those nights

the sky was arctic blue and the land
truly emerald and the town
before it moved upscale was still

in love with itself and all of us above
all else in love with that lunar light

Heather McHugh

FOURTH OF JULY, B. C.

Each evening brings its modicum
of glitter to the nation. But this one is the work
of some uncommon pyrotech: the blue and scarlet biospheres
blown up and then flown off—the people left
in dazzling dandelion-drift . . . by dint of which

the topical becomes the typical again,
the shimmer just a shine. (Did I imagine them?
Those flashy chemistries and colored concentrations
twenty miles across the sea, were thy
just eye-salts, mind-motes, practice
for an aneurysm? Blink, and proud
America comes down

to dust and asterisks.)
But there, above
Port Angeles,
unmoved,

is sheer
Olympic imperturbability—a hundred
times a township's height, an impassivity attended by
impressive skies of its own manufacture. Men had best
beware: the price of its ascent is steep:
the peak of its indifference

is monumental, unrelated to the flags
we've chosen from our local five-and-ten.
The mountain's root is fire;
the mountain's flower is frost:
our thoughts won't keep
inside its ken. A final poof!
and men are scattered

into manyness again . . .

Heather McHugh

IMPOLITIC

Into the soothing sound-proofed hundred-powered
air of SUV and cruise ship cream there comes
the clop of the fetlocked one, the blinked mare, the one

who carriages her way along the docks, past mansioned points
and pollardings of park (in short, wherever seaside seers
may care to steal a scene, or four, or more, for

pocket-cameras; steal an hour, or half,
or less, from pocket-watches, talk
talk talking as they go). But dallying is what she

doesn't do, who has to drag them,
sometimes five or six obesities
down Dallas Road, to where

she's hinted with a whipper's lick
to turn (at Turner: here
the clopping's altered,

clipped, a swift decision
brought to bear—she has to cross
oncoming chrome—a will is rallied,

wherewithal applied.) And then the corner
braved and left behind, the lower
slower pockmarks settle back,

distinctly four,
from which
the balconist's

unholidaying ear picks up
the oddity for which it was alert:
the quirk of individuation, twist

of hand or tendency of hoof,
discernible at last above
the scenic generality:

for one
most clearly (more
than all or some) will hurt.

Heather McHugh

SAMPLING

When the table is turned, the hand
resists: it's a drag—then suddenly

it's a rhythm section. Needlestick of stimulant
for some two-timing touch; a centrifuge for

boost and beat. (It burns to move, it turns the tunes
to hiccup-arts all down the street.) Such feline

felonies! Such licks of scratch!—insinuated
into sitting rooms, where someone's upright

grandma thinks of love—and gets
amen, a mensch, a mention—

(all because bad vinyl snagged
the handyman's attention . . .).

Heather McHugh

BACK TO B.C.

Streaming, striped with
blown snow-smoke, the
highway ran at odds with
wind the whole of Man-
itoba and Saskatchewan.
The trouble was the truck

took broadside dispositions
From the wind; the eye
(which drove the mind's
attention to the road)
was now forever being teased
from its intents and constancies.
otherwise, weatherless, it would
have been at one with all

The strictland flats of Middle West
macadam. Here instead, in twists
and tails, to find its wits consorting
with the mist!—this little was
too much! The brightest roadlines
disappeared.) The mind is made
to discipline the eye so that that the eye
can aim the mind—or else
the troubled vision thinks

I know my own way home, I'll show
these whippersnappers what a looker is . . .).

*

But then the landscape did
let up, its sweep diverted
into big and little vortices by
foothills: dark and highland
sorts of snow

began to dim
the enterprise. The truck's
own motion in the midnight drove,
by pointillistic billions, into eyeshot,
sycophants the host was both
attracting and attracted to.
(Mis-matcher or
mote-mesmerizer,
specialist in quirk,

the mind's impressionism always runs
the risk of masterwork.)

*

You think you're home free,
coasting down the coastal side? Think twice, think more—
no polymath can think enough. The ultimate seduction lies
before you, in a temperate domain,

along a trail you trust, just
hours short of home's familiar shift,

where Sleep Incorporated veers across your path—
to silverize your dust,
to destinize your drift . . .

Don McKay

SONG OF THE SAXIFRAGE TO THE ROCK

Who is so heavy with the past as you,
Monsieur Basalt? Not the planet's most muscular
depressive, not the twentieth century.
How many fingerholds
have failed, been blown or washed away, unworthy
of your dignified *avoirdupois*, your strict
hexagonal heart? I have arrived to show you, first
the interrogative mood, then secrets of the niche,
then Italian. Listen, slow one,
let me be your fool, let me sit
on your front porch in my underwear
and tell you risqué stories about death. Together
we will mix our dust and luck and turn ourself
into the archipelago of nooks and graves.

Don McKay

"STRESS, SHEAR, AND STRAIN THEORIES OF FAILURE"
Charles Nevin, *Principles of Structural Geology*

They have never heard of lift
and are—for no one, over and over—cleft. Riven,
recrystallized. Ruined again. The earth-engine
driving itself through death after death. Strike/slip,
thrust, and the fault called normal, which occurs
when two plates separate.
Do they hearken unto Orpheus, whose song
is said to make them move? Sure.
This sonnet hereby sings that San Fran-
cisco and LA shall, thanks to its chthonic shear,
lie cheek by jowl in thirty million
years. Count on it, mortals. Meanwhile,
may stress shear strain attend us. Let us fail
in all the styles established by our lithosphere.

Don McKay

SPECIFIC GRAVITIES: #76 (MARBLE)

To whom we turn to be
momentous, to be
monumental, to be
meant. As I browse
among the statues it appears
that marble is the way eternity
confers itself on breasts, it seems
that even pubic hair (David's,
for example), if redone in fine Carrara
marble, can become a simulacrum of the absolute
one flare of graven
everliving fire.
                    But then,
on my way home, I take
a shortcut through the graveyard
and get mixed signals from the stones
Are these the sculpted entrances to rooms
(de lux, I guess) located elsewhere?
Or should we think of them as exits—
holes the dead fell through
which we have squared up, plugged, and,
putting the best face upon it,
polished?
                    And this: once
in Limerick, in a tiny tourist trap,
I came upon an egg of Connemara marble.
Heavy in the hand it was,
heavy as an egg whose embryo
foresaw its end, heavy as the one egg laid
by Schopenhauer's chicken. The past perfect
spoke to my fingers, who had fallen for it,
hard. "See that window?
Throw me through it. *Now.*"

Don McKay

ASTONISHED—

astounded, astonied, astunned, stopped short
and turned toward stone, the moment
filling with its slow
stratified time. Standing there, your face
cratered by its gawk,
you might be the symbol signifying aeon.
What are you, empty or pregnant? Somewhere
sediments accumulate on seabeds, seabeds
rear up into mountains, ammonites
fossilize into gems. Are you thinking
or being thought? Cities
as sand dunes, epics
as e-mail. Astonished
you are famous and anonymous, the border
washed out by so soft a thing as weather. Someone
inside you steps from the forest and across the beach
toward the nameless all-dissolving ocean.

George McWhirter

CONVICTION

Like the feet of children tingle
And smart on the shingle,
Whose faces glow and sting
With sun and seaside visiting,

As spiders as green as can be,
On evenings as wide as the sea,
Walk, without the slightest fuss,
In harmony with the octopus

On legs as fine and fair
As baby hair,
Or platinum eyelash
Of the moon, whose light will wash

Over as though the car were coral,
A reef of metal
In the night. Like they breed dilemma
On the radio antenna,

Webbed through the air, the sweet
Music of their feet
Treads into my head
The stickiness of love I dread.

Like them I walk a plank
Of moonlight for my lank
Captaincy of love—old stiff
Transported in a skiff,

Whose oars
Are four
Fingers, and
Hull, a hand

That seeks your face, as if it were Van
Dieman's Land

George McWhirter

ON SENDING OUT OUR KIDS AGAIN

> *"Sugar and spite*
> *make everything night."*

(A plea for an end to child sacrifice to the gods, for Karen Cooper)

Why should we dress them up
and send them out on Sunday
or any other day?

Why should we lay the inverted barnacles
of our children's ears on the rock of ages
to be smashed?

           Be it
the sober grey serge
            of Presbyterian granite. Or Jesuit
obsidian. Or pure Koranic chalk, made from the snow
of protozoa in the Persian Gulf.
                    Or basalt that seeps—to my
 Ulster eye— like O'Neil's blood into the slim strands
of Strangford Lough,
              as rag-endy
                      as the wrist he slashed off
and the hand he flung like a son
ahead of him to touch shore first, telling all
of his immortal will to win
over a Scottish giant
in this wee wager
of an ocean race.)
                  But what can the astonished
gashes of our children's mouths report, but burial? The gags
are these gross convulsions of folded stone
that resemble us in bed,
              which must play

their hard copulations backwards
at minus ten billion motions
to the moment
to get hot
with the engendering
again.
The smile crossing
our children's faces is the cosmic splash, the hit movie
we have waited all of time for at the box-office,
the blockbuster in the Hollywood
on Broadway.
These dimpled chins are not made to be our
  animated glyphs,
our impertinent messages written
into their infant skin
for God, but God's kisses turned into lips that wet our cheeks.
Waddling, falling, gasping, snuffling,
they come asking us
to wipe their noses, change
their sodden socks, un-mummify
them from their muddy-buddies.
Let us get up off our asses and our knees. Find baby Buddha,
Jesus and Mohammed their Huggies.
Stop stuffing their genitals
with gelignite, sending them out
into the street, to knock on our neighbours' doors,
begging for a fistful
of poisoned
Halloween candies
to make their visit worthwhile.

Joseph Millar

GIRLFRIENDS

They come jittering into her life from the past,
brunette like her mother, wiry
and tense, wearing garments the color
of anthracite chopped from the heart
of the city. Complaint rises like music
or smoke past the elegant lamps of their faces
as they settle their black fringe and nail polish
onto our secondhand couch: men, mostly,
but the theme could be anything,
children, money, uterine cramping,
low brilliant choruses of damage and pain.

They tell her their dreams, of roses
and falling. They point to the crow's feet
deepening each year beside
the flat wings of their cheek bones.

In the one painting my mother left
when she died, the waves are breaking
over Folly Cove. All night they will break
in the autumn dark, while one friend sleeps
holding onto her boy-lover and another
drives south through the rain-soaked hills
bound for her sister's third wedding. They
carry the yoke of the city's blue lights
easily back toward morning. They feel
their bodies grow beautiful, the night sky
smoothing their faces and hair. Nobody
needs to tell them death's hands
keep opening over the road.

Joseph Millar

JUNKYARD

Except for the goldenrod covered with dust
and the blue cinders under the tracks,
except for the gondolas loaded with scrap iron
like boxes of flowers unpacked by the dead,
this could be a church for the resurrection
of car thieves past and still serving time.

You can smell gear oil and antifreeze
leeching into the ground. You can see distant
tidal basins glowing like mercury off to the west.
Who will be left to pardon us now, the boy
with crosses tatooed on both hands who rolled
the stripped Thunderbird into the river?

Or the machinist laid off from Bethlehem Steel
caste marks of grease anointing each knuckle,
who hot-wired a Chrysler parked by the gates,
haunted by dreams of cylinders firing, fan blades
leaping free in their shroud, the stopped world looking
up, amazed, stuck like a rock in its own black mud.

Joseph Millar

ELDERS

At the end of December the cold rain blows
on the swaths of fog lying for miles
down the hills and onto the hawk
waiting motionless on his bare branch
furred with lichen. It falls
on the snow geese who press
their breast feathers into the drifted leaves
and onto the tree trimmer hired by the county
who shaves doug fir stobs back to the trunk
so they won't hook the power lines
swaying there over the narrow road.

Once home, I let the two boys
in black suits carrying the Book of Mormon
pray for me right here on the front porch
though I wither some under their fixed, bright gaze.
I'm hoping the tulip bulbs from last fall
have started new roots in the freezing mud,
that the leaf mold heaped along the back fence
will protect the new ferns and bamboo.

Christmas tree skeleton, where did the years
piled on my father's back come from?
I know he never wanted a funeral.
Some mornings I drink coffee for hours
outside the bait shop west of town
where the old men gather to warm themselves,
hat brims low shading their faces,
their lost stories drifting away on the wind.

I want to rest my head on the chest
of the old crab boat skipper
who sighs to himself, watching the harbor
heave and swell, chafing
the fuel dock's hawsers down
before he seats himself in the metal skiff
waiting to be cast off.

Joseph Millar

HANSEL AND GRETEL'S FATHER EXPLAINS

Children, I chose the woman
because she sang in the kitchen
a thin song about the apple harvest
and because her skirts rustled
when she undressed by the window,
a bird of prey in the dark. In spring
she'd bring my lunch to the woods
and sit close on a fallen log, one hand
on my leg, watching me eat. I chose
her red mouth because it promised
secrets I'd dreamed of always:
kissing in the extravagant decay
of an ancient rose arbor, brocade
of black thorns crossing the sky. In winter
the dark flowers her body smelled of
helped me forget the January wind
sharpening itself like an axe blade
over the frozen lake, and the wolves
howling deep in the pines. God
help me, I wanted to sleep forever,
curled up at her feverish breast.
How many times I've followed the path
we took that last day through the trees,
the ravens' iron voices mocking
my shamed flesh. I dreamed I saw
a boy's blond hair matted with blood,
the burned face of a woman seven feet tall,
my crimes like dark sperm blossoms
under her dress. And maybe I've only dreamed
this as well: spring rain in the forest,
new grass in the fields, your hands
holding mine in the uneasy clasp
of childhood's helpless forgiveness.

Susan Musgrave

ORIGAMI DOVE

Every Christmas Eve we would drive
through the ritzy district to see
the coloured lights my father said
were an utter waste of electricity.
He took the long way home, the way
that wound away around the orphanage—
a waste of gas, my mother thought,
but for once didn't say—and I would
imagine, for an instant, a world
where someone is grateful for something.
As we slowed past that desperate house
always in darkness, *those poor bastards*,
my father would say, the pitch of their roof
made it impossible for Santa's reindeer
to land there. At home we'd hang stockings,
leave milk and shortbread by the chimney,
whisper our prayers, and I'd lie awake thinking
what it must feel like to have no one.
Every year my father took the one
trustworthy ladder we owned and climbed high
onto our flat roof and sat drinking
whiskey and ringing bells so we would go on
being deceived as long as it was possible
to go on being children; he knew love
and treachery were part of the same

bargain. Lately I have come to believe
all that is of value is the currency
of the heart, so that when my father
lay dying, I forgave God. I had never believed
in him until then, but found myself
forgiving him for the space he had never filled,
the loneliness in me he had created. Now I know
this: between birth and death there is *only*

loneliness, so big sometimes it makes love
seem spectacularly small, with no grave
big enough to contain our grief. Loneliness

takes the good out of all of our goodbyes,
more permanent than the sadness you know
when your lover drives away having lost
interest in everything about you, especially
your suffering. Love's a blip, a glitch,
but loneliness signs on for the duration,
one gunshot wound to the head is all it takes
to assure your allotted space in today's
News of the World beside the Bangladesh woman
caned 101 times for having an abortion, misery
being careless and everywhere
at the same time. Loneliness is so big

that when he moves into your house you feel
as if someone has moved away, warmed up the Dead
Wagon with one headlight missing
and made for the highway still chasing
love, the thing you both swore you'd always die for.
Now loneliness has laid me instead, lopsided,
on the table, so that when they come to view me,
the one or two people who tried to know me, will say
"She never looked that way, he's got her mouth
all wrong," as if the living shouldn't have to see
how right we finally become. If my mouth looks wrong

it's because I am trying to find the way
to tell you I have become the AIDS baby
who doesn't want to die until she has seen
her first snow, an origami dove
chased by a flying child under a snow-dusted
school bus in Ontario, now buried

a kindly stone's throw from a frozen river.
The cure or loneliness, they say, is solitude,
trust everybody but cut the cards, take your delight
in momentariness, avoid adjectives of scale,
you will love the world more and desire it
less: all sound advice. There are 101 words
for freedom, not one from the kind of pain
the woman must have suffered after 101
lashes with a cane, cut, I suspect,
specifically for one purpose. Sex, death,
our fragile lives are like the knife edge
of the wind scraping away the sky. I see how true
loneliness has become when he takes up with me
and walks me through the world I have always
called my home. Only in darkness I see now
it has never been my home.

Susan Musgrave

THE ROOM WHERE THEY FOUND YOU

smelled of Madagascar vanilla.
After touching you for the last time
I scrubbed the scent from my skin—I would try
to remember later what the water felt like
on my hands but it was like trying to remember
thirst when you are drowning. They say love
doesn't take much, you just have to be there
when it comes around. I'd been there
from the beginning, I've been here all along.

I believed in everything: the hope
in you, your brokenness, the way
you arranged cut flowers on a tray
beside my blue and white teacup, the cracked
cup I'd told you brought me luck, the note
you wrote, "These flowers are a little ragged
—like your husband." The day you died

of an overdose in Vancouver
I found a moonshell in the forest, far
from the sea; when I picked it up
and pressed it to my ear I could hear you
taking the last breath you had the sad luck

to breathe. Our daughter cupped her hands
over her ears, as if she could stop death
from entering the life she had believed in
up until now. Childhood, as she had
known it, was over: the slap
of the breakers, the wind bruising the sea
tells her she is no longer safe in this world—

it's you she needs. I see you pulling away
after shooting up in the car while we
stood crying on the rain-dark road,
begging you to come home. The vast sky
does not stop wild clouds
from flying. This boundless grieving,
for whom is it carried on?

Susan Musgrave

OUT OF TIME

Who plans it, whoever looks
up at the stars the first time
and thinks they've seen it all.
Same thing, night after night. Nothing
astonishes them. No, the first time
you look at the stars you think
you, too, could live forever. You're parked
in the van, a babyseat in the back,
smoking your own brand, drinking
white wine from the bottle while he points out
the Big Dipper, the Milky Way
before slipping a condom over the tip
of his service revolver and forcing it
down your throat. The stars blank out
one by one as he starts to push
harder on the back of your head, spinning
the barrel, thinking because you let him
pick you up it meant you wanted to go
even further. "I'll make you a star,"
he says, pulling back on the hammer;
you're running out of breath.
He lights his last cigarette
and you relive forever in that
moment, waiting for the click.

P. K. Page

From HAND LUGGAGE—A MEMOIR IN VERSE

Calgary. The twenties. Cold and the sweet
melt of chinooks. A musical weather.
World rippling and running. World
watery with flutes. And woodwinds.
The wonder of water in that icy world.
The magic of melt. And the grief of it. Tears—
heart's hurt? heart's help?

This was the wilderness: western Canada.
Tomahawk country—teepees, coyotes,
cayuses and lariats. The land that Ontario
looked down its nose at. Nevertheless
we thought it civilized. Civilized? Semi.

Remittance men, ranchers—friends of my family—
public school failures, penniless outcasts,
bigoted bachelors with British accents.
But in my classroom, Canadian voices—
hard r's and flat a's, a prairie language
—were teaching me tolerance, telling me something.
This vocal chasm divided my childhood.
Talking across it, a tightrope talker,
corrected at home, corrected in classrooms:
wawteh, wadder—the wryness of words!

Such my preparation for a life of paradox—
a borderland being, barely belonging,
one on the outskirts, over the perimeter.

I was deceptive, full of disguises
a poet in residence, a private person
masked as a malamute—mutable, moody—
but would dance on a table, or argue the dawn up—
a jack-in-the-box, 'a jolly good sport'.

Tennis or riding—you'd only to try me.
The smell of a loose-box—of straw and manure
ammonia, saddle-soap, hay, the metallic
jingle of bridles, 'Gear, tackle and trim',
wild roses and lupins—sweetscent of the prairies.

Greys, dapples, and sorrels, bays, chestnuts and pintos—
I rode them and loved them. Their rumps were French polished
their noses were velvet, wet velvet their mouths.
But fording a river, face into the current,
they were Poseidon's. Hooves slipping and sliding
flesh plunging and rising, they struggled and swam.

And so, I suppose, I struggled and swam
because where I was centred, what mattered, was art—
the pre-Raphaelites, Rodin and Renoir and Rouault
el Greco and Epstein, Picasso, Van Gogh—
I cherished them all in their cheap reproductions.

And poems. The pattern of vowels in a poem
the clicking of consonants, cadence, and stress—
were magic and music. What matter the meaning?
The sound was the meaning—a mantra, a route
to the noumenon, not that I'd thought
that through absolute pitch I'd re-pattern myself.
What I'd thought? What I'd felt. For me feeling was thinking.
I thought with my heart—or so my heart thought.

P. K. Page

AH, BY THE GOLDEN LILIES

> *. . . ah by the golden lilies,*
> *the tepid, golden water,*
> *the yellow butterflies*
> *over the yellow roses . . .*
> —*Yellow Spring Juan Ramón Jiménez*

Jiménez, but for the roses
you paint a Rio garden
where every golden morning
the golden sunlight spills
on my Brazilian breakfast—
coffee like bitter aloes
strawberry-fleshed papayas
the sensuous persimmon . . .
My young head full of follies
ah, by the golden lilies.

Beneath the cassia boughs
where fallen yellow blossoms
reflect a mirror image
I barefoot in the petals
trample a yellow world
while small canaries flutter
over the lotus pond.
I trail my golden fingers—
for I am Midas' daughter—
in the tepid, golden water.

My blue and gold macaw
laughs his demented laughter
dilates his golden pupils—
a golden spider spins
a spangled golden web
for beauty-loving flies.

Above the cassia branches—
the cassia colored sun.
Above the yellow lilies—
the yellow butterflies.

Jiménez, I am freed
by all this golden clangor.
Jiménez, your roses
denote a falling sound
a sound that will not rhyme
with *sambas jocosos*
macumba, feijoada
Bahían *vatapá.*
A different sun disposes
over the yellow roses.

Suzanne Paola

THE SECOND LETTER OF ST. PAUL ON THE HUMAN GENOME PROJECT

I sound harder on you than I mean—
you never did anything but what your forty-six chromosomes
cried out for, in their carhorn piston voices.
Up where I am we can hear them, 4 billion of you
& the rauc rising: more & more.
From the first murder, gentle Neanderthal (Abel)
slaughtered by Homo sapiens (Cain). You did
what we asked you to do.
We put mammals in front of your eyes
& you switched from grasses to meat, cheek teeth
sunk like medieval towers crumbled
in the Age of Reason. As soon as you knew
fire you fire-hunted, burning forests to take the few
whatever that might run out to you.
You've never been gentle, is what I mean, & your gentler nature
you forget as quickly as your gods. Whom you make,
slap into the sky & then let fall.
"Prophets have never enjoyed a Darwinian
edge," the biologist said, & those of us here can't pull you out
anymore, of your bodies; you've mapped them well, & you
love those twists & ends.

Suzanne Paola

PATIENT 6

*From August 1946 to January 1947, the University of Rochester
conducted toxicity studies on uranium, using hospital patients as
subjects. Highly enriched uranium (uranium-234 and uranium-
235) was administered intravenously.*
  —*Department of Energy Roadmap Human Radiation Experiments*

Studies, Investigation, Research

The premise of science: There must be more.
The premise of art: There must be more.
The premise of history: More. More. More.

Deep in this brief & unsupportive body
where dissectors' knives first parsed the slub & ooze,
the sacs where blood's squeezed, the lobes
where fluid taints or air's thinned or.
Or. What goes in
comes out stripped, stinking.

In the Renaissance the body's back
as Idea. It's still soul they seek, that second appendix,
slack bag waiting for the immaculate invisible to come.

*What the body consumeth cannot be said
to profit thereby*

one dissector writes, sick
with the carnival tangle of intestine & that's
disappointing but not too terribly (there's More)
in the cardiocentric or craniocentric body (nobody's sure
where soul's couched). Leonardo
sketching the optic nerves, almost
as an afterthought.

The search is on. Some cadavers
coming to the dissecting table oddly gouged & warm.

Suzanne Paola

HP6

The purpose of the studies was to determine the dose level at which renal injury is first detectable . . . Human subjects included four males and two females, all with good kidney function, ranging in age from 24 to 61 years.

All had medical conditions, such as undernutrition, alcoholism, or heart disease.

Flash. Dr. Samuel Bassett's "production
line" (he calls it). He searches
ERs at Christmas to keep the holidays from slowing him.
Looking for the subjects he calls, for the experiment,
Human Products: HP1, HP2, HP3 . . .
The point (More): to see how much radioisotope
the human kidney holds.

("He was not a ghoul," Dr.
Patricia Durbin said. "He was a scientist.")

The HPs hallucinating, malnourished, good enough.
HP (Patient) 6 he-who-gets-most
at 71 micrograms per kilo, up from the 6
where Bassett started

to find that dose of soluble uranium salt which, when introduced intravenously as a single dose, would produce just detectable

renal injury

Greg Pape

FOUR SWANS

A northern harrier glides low over the tules.

A pair of mallards, their tail feathers
tipped up to the sun, feed in what's left
of the open water on Whistler Pond.

January. Four white tundra swans
stand at the edge of the ice.

Grace. Peace. Dignity. X.

X stretches her long gorgeous neck,
steps off the ice onto the water
and keeps walking.

When I spoke on the phone with my mother
in the hospital, someone was dying

in the background. I imagined hope
dripped from a pouch into a tube
into a vein. A moan

took off and scaled up into a scream.
I can't talk, my mother said, firmly,
and there at the margins of her voice

some hard anger pushed against terror.
Pain sat and watched.

Now I sit and watch the swan
walk on water. There must be

a shelf of ice just under the surface.

She lowers herself, and with a twitch
of her tail feathers, pushes off
and glides into the open water,

not like the setting out at the beginning
of a story, more like easing into

a new stillness, this white house of down
and feathers from which the ripples
move outward, signals from a beacon,

but at the same time appear
to move inward, drawn, repelled and drawn.

I see a boy drawn to the window
of the last house on Congress Street,
the small white adobe at the foot
of Tumamoc Hill in Tucson. He is

looking at the full moon
through bare branches of the Palo Verde tree,
imagining the body spread-eagle, caught

in flight by those branches
a dozen yards from the spot Joe Galindo's
motorcycle hit the wall at sixty.

To him Galindo is a story told by the neighbors,
a cautionary tale of speed and booze
and reckless disregard.

To him Galindo is a moonlit thought
tangled in the limbs among his own
confusions, a ghost among other ghosts,

only this one the closest, the one that holds sway
between the Palo Verde and the small cave
in the hillside where the plaster statue

of Saint Jude resides. Maybe X
I should name Saint Jude, patron saint of the X's.

She feeds on the pond bottom
with the mallards.

She works her black feet back and forth
in the bottom-mud stirring things up

then lowers her long neck in a bow
and dips her head into the water.

Miranda Pearson

THE EMPRESS

Naked
on an unmade bed   a mermaid on a rock
          she can hear
the seagull's throaty cry   dumb and erotic
and all around
the deep boom of the hotel, its heart-
beat.

She's floating on the bed, an island
in this chintz room she hired,
          each room
a cell in the hive.

No one knows she's here
it's like a death
an erasure
a field of snow
(she stays away from the window, believes
in the pull   in sudden helplessness).

The hotel
is dressed in ivy and ivory
a desiccated tiger
rears over the fireplace, snarling and flattened

the ping   of the elevator
the surprise of it opening and who
might be standing there   she is

a woman   toppling into middle age
she is   the fat lady in the mirror
resigned to the fuggish clan of her body, its
ordinary secrets

she is   eating birthday cake (a small
silver fork)   her brain's intestines
closely packed   a knot of thought
a flock of naught

flock vines climb the walls   she wonders
          if she has been greedy, like the British Museum,
collected more
than she needed.

Past lovers swarm   like military elite, like
ground cover—sometimes she'd like to return
all the artefacts, all the relics.

One true thing: *la jouissance*—the mother-bliss
she has known that (and what I say
is the truth and only the truth so help me God).

Along *The Shining* corridors
hang sepia photographs: Big ships
  plough their way into this land

beyond velvet drapes   pink flowers read
     Welcome To Victoria
Up close they're pink flowers
up close   she is mired
a mother   her smothering skirts
(*mère   mer*   the sea
                    of the body)

up close she is cranky w/frown lines
vain and depressive   she is
forty
cosseted by heredity   eating cake
secrets fizzing in her blue veins
in her wrists
her shaking hands.

Today   happiness is
tended silence, the hotel room's isolation tank
a port
neither here   nor there

the small ship of cake is a pretty thing,
its strata of red gel, its snowy glaze

she is not (at heart) a femme, her elegance
            imported, misfit,
but she can't help
her hugely soft female body
and she has always loved lilies
their thick scent, their staining hearts

all the interior spaces of femininity:
the parlours   the dining rooms   the gardens
she ponders them
            in her heart.

The past
            streams out behind her
its terrible flare
Isadora's scarf   tangled in the wheels.

In this new country
she loves the log booms   those gatherings
of past lives
jostling and waiting, how they
hitch together   how they
unhook—

but still   she is hostage to Wordsworth
the chiffon mist
the cold sweat of dew

to the dark topiary at Hever, the carp
that slowly patrol the moats.

             Nostos   *isn't cricket—that dreary paradigm of death.*
Isn't   teashops   tins of tea   Harrods   Christ! All that,

it's the gestures
the hats   frozen in the air: goodbye
goodbye   *I'm gone*   *I'm gone*   *I'm gone*   *I'm gone*   *I'm*

It's the white iris bulbs she smuggled over, wrapped in muslin
struggled to replant (pathetic
trying to re-create Sissinghurst on a six foot square balcony)

that narrative embarrasses her now
her privileged story of loss
seems juvenile, sentimental
         yet

it's the balm that makes sense
gives reason

to fetish

to the pink ribbon around the love letters
the photographs
the pressed flowers

those small ruins   where memory stays

where happiness is dust, a bouquet   a thrown hat.

Love,   spread thick   its lovely
                              glaze—

Peter Pereira

ANAGRAMMER

If you believe in the magic of language,
then *Elvis* really *Lives*
and *Princess Diana* foretold *I end as car spin.*

If you believe the letters themselves
contain a power within them,
then you understand
what makes *outside tedious,*
how *desperation* becomes *a rope ends it.*

The circular logic that allows *senator* to become *treason,*
and *treason* to become *atoners.*

That *eleven plus two* is *twelve plus one,*
and an *admirer* is also *married.*

That if you could just re-arrange things the right way
you'd find your true life,
the right path, the answer to your questions:
you'd understand how *the Titanic*
turns into *that ice tin,*
and *debit card* becomes *bad credit.*

How *listen* is the same as *silent,*
and not one letter separates *stained* from *sainted.*

Peter Pereira

THE DEVIL'S DICTIONARY OF MEDICAL TERMS

—after Ambrose Bierce, 1842–1914

Allergies: Large lies. Eager ills.
Antibiotics: Is it botanic?
Antidepressant: President Satan.
Appendicitis: Septic 'n' I paid.
C-section: Nice cost.
Chronic Fatigue Syndrome: Oh, my secure grand fiction!
Depression: Snide poser. Person dies.
Dementia: I'd eat men. Detain me.
Dermatitis: Am dirtiest.
Diabetes Mellitus: Diet abuses met ill.
Erectile Dysfunction: Lucifer's indecent toy.
Flatulence: Clean flute.
Gastroenteritis: Rattiest regions.
Gall stones: Lost angels.
Heart Attacks: That's a racket.
Hepatitis: I spit hate.
Hypertension: Shy inner poet.
Lower Back Pain: Incapable work.
Manic Depressive: Impressive dance.
Migraine: I'm in rage.
Neurotic: Unerotic.
Night Sweats: Things waste.
Nocturnal Enuresis: Encounters urinals. In unclean trousers.
Prostate Cancer: Crap! Not as erect. Procreates? Can't.
Renal Failure: Funereal lair.
Surgery: Guys err.
Tension Headache: Death's inane echo.
Uterine Prolapse: Plenteous repair.
Vasectomy: My octaves!
Whiplash Injury: Shh! I win jury, pal.
X-ray Department: Darn pretty exam.
Yeast Vaginitis: It's a nasty I give.
Zoonotic Diseases: Societies and zoos.

Lucia Perillo

FOR THE FIRST CROW WITH WEST NILE VIRUS TO ARRIVE IN OUR STATE

For a long time you lay tipped on your side like a bicycle
but now your pedaling has stopped. Already
the mosquitoes have chugged their blisterful of blood
and flown on. Time moves forward,
no cause to weep, I keep reminding myself of this:
the body will accrue its symptoms. And the grammar books,
which tell us not to use the absolutes, are wrong:
the body will always accrue its symptoms.

But shouldn't there also be some hatchlings within view:
sufficient birth to countervail the death?
At least a zero on the bottom line:
I'm not asking for black integers,
just for nature not to drive our balance into the dirt.

Unless Darwin was wrong about those Galapagosian finches.
The bird-books give us mating calls but not too many death-songs.
And whereas the Jews have their Kaddish and the Tibetans
have their strident prayers, all I have is sweet talk
for the barricades of heaven. Where you, my vector,
soar already, a sore thumb amongst the clouds.

Still in the denuded maple I can see one of last year's nests
waiting to be filled again, a ragged mass of sticks.
Soon the splintered shells will fill it
as your new geeks claim the sky, I guess in any
burgling of the bloodstream, something yolky has to break.
And I write this as if language could restitute the breakage—
or make you lift your head from its quilt of wayside trash.
Or retract the mosquito's proboscis, but that's language again,
whose five-dollar words not even can unmake you.

Lucia Perillo

VIAGRA

"Let the dance begin."

In magazine-land, you two are dancing—
though a moment ago you were engaged
in some activity like stringing fenceline
or baling hay—why else the work gloves
sticking up from your back pockets?
In a whirlwind of pollen, you-the-man
have seized the urge to gather you-the-woman
to your breast—his breast, her breast, tenderly, tenderly—
now you turn away and shyly grin.
Oh you possessors of youthful haircuts
& attractive activewear from L.L. Bean,
you who have the still small-enough asses
to permit the rearview photograph:
don't you already have enough silver pouring
from life's slot? But no, you also want
the river's silver surge where its bed drops off,
you want the namesake in all its glory—*Niagra*:
even with the barge of animals teetering on its lip.
This ploy was wrought by some 19th century huckster,
the honeymooners gathered on the shore's high bank
to watch the barge drop as the creature-cries* rise up . . .
before all the couples re-cottage themselves
to do what, then what, it's hard to imagine
after so much death. I always thought *Tigers*
until I read the barge was full of dgos and cats—
one baby camel, a demented old monkey,
le petit-mort, that little French whimper
given up by the ordinary before it crashes into splinters.
So the widow Taylor straps herself in a barrel
and rides it safely over the century's cusp,
& Maud Willard imbarrels herself with her dog
who'll leap from the busted staves alone.

Still, wouldn't the ride be worth that one live leap—
doesn't part of us *want* to broken to bits?
After all, our bodies are what cage us,
what keep us, while, outside, the river
says more, wants more, is more: the *R*
(*grrrr, argh, graa . . .) in all its variegated coats.
A sound always coming, always smashing, always spoken
by the silver teeth and tongue that fill the river's open throat.

Paulann Petersen

VOLUPTUARIES

The earth flicks, twirls
the feathery torque of its growth.
Evened spaces fall down, shatter,
scatter away, the ratchet of birdsong
repleting. To then pause, repeat.

Passing through what might be
inclined to throw down a shadow,
light becomes wings so yellow
they're breathless, blades
so quick and thin they sing.

Air shimmies outward, gold shinnies
up the trees. A perfume brews
for drinking—long gulps,
deep drafts. Liquor of pollen,
ester of want and plenty.

The weighty, suffusing, never-to-be
satisfied. With vernal string
wafted from green, leaf-ladders
braid themselves up and into
the somewhere of blue.

Steven Price

APOLOGIA PRO VITA SUA

I, too, would wish to write otherwise.
In any age it is shameful to write
of men and yet more shameful not to.
Still language conspires, forgets man
is a cavity in a skull, meat-tongued, fleshy,
little else. Our bodies mostly hymns to pain,
as if a strop of butcher knives, of blood-
knotted leather might lead us nearer God.
The saints dreamed it: any cruelty done
upon us can as surely be done by us.
And is. Forgive us our faith in steel, muscle,
the mud-crusted, too-human boot. What use
are words at such an hour? In Tehran,
roped to his chair, did the poet Baraheni
admire his own cries? Feet splitting like figs
in seed. A second, barbed scream inside him
of his own making.

Steven Price

UPON THE DELIBERATION OF THEIR DOMESTIC POLICY

At last they passed the motion that death, being an infringement upon the basic dignities of man, be cast out in exile and spurned with the full force of the law. There was a general shuffling of papers, a dry cough or two, the crossing and uncrossing of trousers, but the act itself was astonishingly simple to put through. A dignitary from the territories stood to assure the members that death would find no refuge in the north. Each of the ten provinces unveiled a plan for the purging of borders. Special interest leaders voiced their assent and swore death in no form allied itself with their movements. It seemed all were in agreement. Death would hereby hold no status, receive no official support, all of its assets and holdings were to be seized immediately and returned to the people. In recognition of this accomplishment the members voted themselves a minor pay increase and declared that day the first day of summer, which it was not, and a day of grand reflection and fine moment, which it was. There followed a great creaking of chairs and shaking of hands. All of this was performed according to the standards of ordinary courtesy and efficiency, as all extraordinary acts of goodness are.

Jarold Ramsey

PENMANSHIP

Squinting at the atrocious scrawl on this page
you might not believe that I was the Penmanship Champion
of the third grade—not for mere handwriting, mind you,
but the pure Art of the Pen, as canonized
long ago by Mr. Palmer and Mr. Rice.
Nobody could touch me when I dipped

my #7 nib in Parker's Quink
and warmed to my left-handed task
of "school figures" first, great stylized L's
and O's and M's looping across the page
much larger and better than life;
and then, best of all, the free exercises

liberated from the ABC's: running helixes,
both conical and cylindrical, clockwise and counter;
bold strokings above and below the line
like a runaway seismograph rewriting
the Richter Scale; and *ne plus ultra*,
the Propeller Series, the very sign of infinity

in motion, my black blades whirling and slicing
stroboscopically on paper always too small
for my flights. Oh, I was the Sonia Heine
and the Igor Sikorsky of the freed pen,
and to be called back to the grubby toolchest
of the alphabet and words cobbled in cursive—

No wonder I scrawl
No wonder I blot

Carlos Reyes

EVERYTHING IS A METAPHOR

for Jonathan Johnson

Outside the cabin: wind, rain drenching
the grass, the trees, a roar waking me
is rushing water of a narrow creek
pulled swifty downhill by its gradients
down to Clark's Fork village
Each pine
needle but a leaf
each wet blade
only grass, yes
each stone slab a step down
but leading only to a mossy lane
A retaining wall
holds but empty shoulder
high iron restraining rings
nothing more sinister
than tethers for mules
their hoof prints long erased
by rain, their steaming breath
dissipated to mist
above the trees

Katrina Roberts

SKIN

A man, an animal, an almond, all find
maximum repose in a shell—so said

Gaston Bachelard. Blame it on the wind.
Blame it on the fog. Eve says, *don't*

change. But how can I not, shot through
as night sky quivering from a star's hurl?

We were just girls together really. I was
wearing it comfortably and it fit. A

neighbor suddenly finds herself allergic
not only to wine but to water—hives

and a closed throat. Llamas scream all
night at the coyotes. You could say I'm

more cauldron than cross. Snakes slink
it off like a diamond-backed argyle sock.

Katrina Roberts

HUNGER

On fishing-line, a nest dangles from a gnarled limb.
In six months' time there will be apples to fill

arms. Where did birds find this filament? Such
active circling and weaving; the dervish love calls

into being . . . How many eggs hatched? How many
did the cats poach, poised as they are to pounce—

orchard their stalking ground? Wing and fur. This
morning: another gopher, its entrails a smear across

the stoop; yesterday, a good-sized quail, dismantled
like a duster, but wet and plump and warm in a

feline mouth. How ravenous they are, essing our legs
in eights—he, with a hunk gouged from his silver

haunch, snagged on a barbed fence, bits of tape-
worm stuck to the plush beneath his upswept tail.

Stan Sanvel Rubin

DOOR

> *"War Dims Hope For Peace"*
> *—from 2004's Best (Actual) Headlines*

It's inevitable, isn't it, that the bulb
in the bathroom is still on
when you go to bed exhausted,
that, slipping between cool sheets,
you can see the phosphorescent lines
of a doorway lit from within,
the blinding outline of light
etching itself into your retina
like an image from Hiroshima

so that you cannot sleep, try as you
might, you cannot close
your eyelids tight enough
to pretend it isn't there,
that thin sketch of illuminated shadow
like rice paper burning,
that patch of nothing suddenly beckoning
through nothing, that hole
in the night, that other doorway.

Stan Sanvel Rubin

MAN ON DECK

This ship is important to him
because somewhere in its lower depths
he hears the sound of his own breathing
as an engine clanking, clanking,
driving the ship on, all the gears grinding,
expenditure of force making
a hash of noise so that he cannot
hear himself think for more than a second
unless he looks beyond the shape of starlit waves
to the wide sea without edges

where, standing and staring there
like a sea-bird born to the sea
with the whole world its circumference,
oblivious to the challenge of fire
because in its dancing it is fire,
he forgets the sounds under his feet,
the skeletal pipes and funnels and valves,
the maze of mechanical accomplishment
that run invisibly everywhere and remembers
the feeling of first voyage, the shore he has left.

Vern Rutsala

TRAVELLING ONE WAY

Sit and listen
              the little towns
call you
         with their dinky stores
and their young evaporating
in summer heat
             between
the angled cars
            moth-wish
and murder mingling some
strangled milkshake
of speed and lassitude
in their blood
            Listen hard
and aim toward
              those towns
the freeway sidesteps
to make them feel bad
about themselves
             Your town is
there somehwere
           lost in maps'
crazy folds
But don't push it
Go town by town
Gather each lost street
in your skimpy harvest
              all those
secret people
          the ghosts you're sure
you know
          before they disappear
squeezed
         to snapshot size

by the rearview mirror
Hear the buzz all things once had
fence wires taut
as banjo strings
    Your town
can't have learned a disguise
good enough to fool you
You know
    every sidewalk crack
that squinting
     angle of the sun
blaring across the lake
that lapping sound
     of water
that pulls a memory
part way out
    then snaps it twanging
back
  skimming the midnight
moontrack toward oblivion
Tonight
   you need the right
names on the right corner
the dog that knows you
and that thin
    volcanic air
that lets you breathe
     again
Pay no attention
to the bum steers
    the rich
dark gives you
    counting its money

And if you play it right
other late ghosts
will turn up
                    paper thin
jogging the road's shoulder
They'll lead you
Call them by name
                        tamarack
fir
   jackpine
              Like whispering
road signs they'll
                    guide you
past moth-wish and murder
along that last sure path
held in place
                  by moon-spattered
lashes of leaves
Just through there your
town waits
              the right names
gathered on the corner
the good dog that knows you
and that ozone air
that teaches you
how to breathe again

Vern Rutsala

LOOKING FOR WORK

Today the line at the soup kitchen
was longer than last week—winter
is coming—and I remember that
summer years ago I spent mornings
on a bench at Third and Salmon
reading the way a hungry man eats,
caught in the gap between two fears—
not finding a job and finding one.
Those fears made the words glow
with extra meaning—I was reading
Lie Down in Darkness and I sank
lower each day into darkness,
the summer slipping away with each
click of the checkers the players
near me moved with such care.
But I couldn't move as if fastened
there reading the same sentence over
and over, lost in a kind of waking coma.
I remember the dusty taste of those
mornings among the old men sunning
their drunk-tank stubble and how I
couldn't walk the block and a half
to the employment office. I knew
nothing waited there but the clerk's
dry lips saying "sorry" or, worse,
offering something terrible, some
blacking factory where I would disappear
forever, eaten alive by America's
fierce indifference. And I was helpless,
holding the book like a life preserver,
knowing I was wholly useless with hands
unable to do anything worth a single
measly dime to anyone anywhere.

Jay Ruzesky

NEW GOD

This time around we're going to make
God out of something a little more
substantial; no more messing with
wisps of smoke, or pillars of light. Let's
use steel or concrete or some of that stuff
NASA uses to keep the space shuttle from
burning up when it hits the atmosphere. Let's
build a big God, higher than the CN tower, so
we can see God for miles and miles. Forget
"God is all around us"; when someone
struggles with ontological angst and wonders
"Where is God in this cruel, cruel world?" we'll
be able to say "Right over there, Dummy." We
could add some more features to God, practical
things: a tire jack, bookshelves, a corkscrew so
if you take a bottle of wine on a picnic but forget
the opener, you won't have to worry. Imagine
living in a world like that.

Ralph Salisbury

MEDICINE-MEETING, HOOPA, 1994

for Helen and Chad

Telling the gathering I'm Cherokee—

    my skin, like the skins
    of many of them, the skin
    of soldiers who tore
    futures not rightfully theirs
    from the genes of defeated populations—

my answers are Father's mother's: "Sassafras tea
for congested lungs; mint leaves
for troubled digestion; willow bark chewed
for pain; tobacco breathed,
into aching ears—"

    and words of love,
    to raise the dead

    in children's dreams
    of living as women and men.

Ralph Salisbury

WE KNEW THEM

Nothing is
particular here. Red—not of
Indian skin
or roses—edges what could be
anyone's garden's
east and west and, then,
back into blackness again, and all
we care for,
a scar's pale summer-lightning on
a graceful knee
in a motel neoned like a hot-day-drink
in, maybe, Ohio—and bandaged,
when tiny, by somebody big—all moves,
like a vivid flock south—
or north—and

We knew them, we say,
knew names from a book between aardvark's
exploring nose and zoo's
zeroes shaped
like Columbus' propped eggs—

knew war-bonnet-feathers that flamed
and warmed us,
from scalp-locks' tousles to
chill-blained,
wornout-moccasin-encumbered,
stubbed toes.

BUCKET

of ashes, the oak,
the maple, heart of the cherry,
red grain of the fir, all burned to drift,
in the bucket I carry. The big dog
is in her small box on top of the piano,
stray bits of bone, ashes, my father too,
among thousands
of white markers. My ashes,
the mark on my forehead made by the thumb
when I kneel by the stove, what
I take away, tend, last night's coals
left to stand in the rain. Nothing tethered now,
char on wind, not the hammered gold leaf
or a vest of stars, not Piaf or Schubert
or poor Balthazar, the mule whose sorry life
was given only to labor, these ashes, my bucket.

Maxine Scates

VICE

When the waiter brought the almond liquor
as courtesy to our table,

I hesitated, remembering Augustine's sin,
the one rewarded by nothing,

neither the delicious anticipation
nor the fall. But the fragrance of a flowering

orchard told me my sin would be rewarded
if I took my first drink in twenty years,

and even as my chorus chattered,
did the work I'm too lazy to do—

this one hates me because I'm a drunk;
this one forgives and says I sought the spiritual

in the spirit's clear distillation; and this one
suggests the timing is right—I knew enough

to know they all could be wrong. And when
I reread Augustine just now, I found

how much I'd misremembered. As a boy,
he'd stolen pears fit only for pigs, yet ate them

anyway. He wanted to taste forbidden fruit
and so did I. My almost sin lived

for its moment with the ringing bells, wild
horses and lush tremolos accompanying a fall.

But when the music faded, I saw
two of us were there—

me and you, the one I will not hurt,
who drank my flowering orchard for me.

Peter Sears

HIGH IN THE BAMBOO

The cat likes to sit in the bamboo,
rest its head on it front paws,
and look out at the world.

I like to sit on the porch,
rest my head against the back of my old chair,
and watch the cat look out at the world.

I look up into the bamboo, too,
glance back down at the cat
to see if it has moved.

It hasn't. I try to catch the cat moving
I don't succeed. I squint to pretend
I am falling asleep. I fall asleep.

When I awake, the cat is gone.
I look back up into the bamboo.
The bamboo tops move.

Tom Sexton

ON THE EMPIRE BUILDER HEADING WEST

On the night after we left Chicago,
Mennonite farmers were ready to step down
at Minot when the train began to slow.
A stranger said that they follow the harvest
until their brethren's fields are chaff and husk
as if time were somehow divisible by grace.
How odd it was that the women's white
bonnets seemed so much whiter in the dark
as a constellation first seen at dusk
seems to deepen with the coming on of night.
We watched them move away from the station
beneath a cloudless sky that promised frost
while we paced and paced, waiting to move on
to Montana and the Cascades by dawn.

Peggy Shumaker

SWANS, WHERE WE DON'T EXPECT THEM

Chena River, Fairbanks

Tundra swans twine necks
among snowflakes
vanishing into evening's

river. Past break up,
tablecloths of rotten ice
nest along the bank.

Halfway, swan wings
open, then settle in
like second thoughts.

Maybe they flew
north over Minto,
traced halos

over brooding ponds,
saw from far up
without touching

the world is hard
and will stay hard
a while longer.

Martha Silano

THE FORBIDDEN FRUIT

was probably an apricot
but is almost always depicted

as shiny and red, the tree
the barren woman's supposed

to roll around beneath,
wash her hands with its juice.

How like us to choose,
for our eye-opening snack,

the one that hybridizes
with any other *Malus*, so that

planting a seed from a small and sour
might well yield a large and sweet.

"A good year for apples,
a good year for twins,"

The Dictionary of Superstitions said,
though weren't we glad when it turned out

not to be true. At the turn of the century,
Tobias Miller brought to Gold Hill, Oregon,

the King, the Northern Spy, the Yellow Transparent,
the Gravenstein, and the Greening,

though we're not sure what we're gathering—
stripy reds we peel and core for sauce,

yellows blushing in the summer sun.
When they ate of it, it tasted good,

twice as good, as say, eternity,
which could not be folded into cake,

which could not be put up or pressed.

Floyd Skloot

GAUGUIN IN OREGON

"Nature is mysteriously infinite and has great powers of imagination."
—*Paul Gauguin*

In relapse again, I have been dreaming
of my body buried in white blossoms
that flutter from the bitter cherry,

soft as the spring breeze and scent
of hyacinth wafting through the screen,
accompanied by a sound like the strokes
of a brush on canvas.
                              An owl?
Deer browsing the hillside trails.
No, the winter creek still surging.

I think I am awake now.
                              Between rains,
finespun mist drifts among the oak
and swaying fir, a ballet choreographed
in dreamtime, costumed in black
and gray. The music, I realize, is made
from shades of dawn, is all cloud,
delicate as the creamy crown
of an early daffodil.
                              My eyes close again,

but then I see him move.
                              Gauguin!
I would know him anywhere. My size,
my age, but looking fresh from a wrestle
with angels. I was reading about him
only yesterday.

          Saffron-colored shirt
like a glimpse of sun, fringe of hair tangling
where I thought to see leaves, bandy legs
unsteady on the sloping land, he reaches
as if grasping one last fruit of the dark.
Where his stained hands slash through a web
of clouds, colors bleed together, stars vanish.

He radiates rage. I sit up against the headboard,
blinking, naked in a snarl of white sheets.
I know I am awake now.
               His form tells me
Gauguin expects to find himself again
in an island paradise. The sort of place,
he wrote, where Life is singing and loving.
The afterlife as advertised to the child
he was in Peru, as dreamed by the seaman
he became in the frozen north, as sketched
by the heartsick wild-man dying on Dominique.
A century dead, he must be more sensitive
to cold than ever. Surely he knows by now
that paradise is approximate.
              Though he lusts
for heat and seething tropical morning light,
here those vapors dancing before his eyes
will have to do. He stalks his way east
toward the crest, lush with Turk's lily
and wild iris. Their sudden color stops him.

Gauguin, if I am not mistaken, is hearing
inner music, a vibration of blues and golds,
the pure vermilion resonance he remembers
as the color a cello turns when played
in its deepest register. I see the savage

glee in his eyes as he looks around,
forgetting where he is in time
to find the lone lilac about to bloom.

Thirst stirs in him. Hunger.
                                    He died
at fifty-five, dreaming of food and wine,
and I am fifty-five, dreaming of burial
by fruit trees that bear no fruit.
Lost in time, back in bed since the dead
of winter, I have woken in the dark
in absolute certainty that it was seven
years ago. Then, in a heartbeat, five
years from now.
                          I must walk to Gauguin
before he vanishes. Against a hazing sky,
he is already growing light and I go out
where the morning colors gather.

Floyd Skloot

BRAHMS IN DELIRIUM

—Vienna, 1890

He hears the sound of sunset as a cello
and snowflakes as flutes above a soft wind
of clarinets. All the reds and yellows
of a fall afternoon are oboes in his mind.

He knows he is out of his mind. He hears
the swift percussion of his racing heart
and feels it carry him toward what he fears
most, the end of all his music, the start

of everlasting silence. Faint harp notes
burst to the surface of each breath. He strips
to the waist, crosses the room. His face floats
in the washstand's mirror and water drips

down his flushed cheeks, his beard. He sees
an overturned jug hover above his head.
Now all it holds are a few melodies,
a passage in strings for all the unsaid

words, a theme shredded like winter light
as the snow ceases to fall. Then, nothing.
Silence will at last fill the room, and night
come on with its own secret songs to sing.

Esta Spalding

THE KEY

While the men in the office continue their never-ending
    deconstruction of Scorcese, she
takes the key from where it hangs, on the hook &
    goes down the hall to the women's washroom—
the one next door to the Birthright clinic where girls who
    have read the ads in buses Pregnant? Need
Help? leave with a stuffed bunny for the baby—& she unbuttons
    wool pants, letting her stomach expand completely for
the first time all morning. Then pushing her cotton panties
    down, she sits on the toilet—institutional, like the
toilets in hospitals—& bleeds.
    They have told her this only means the child
is threatened. Like weather, the pain is
    coming now, building at the base of her back, rolling
up her spine & off her shoulders, so she leans
    her head between her knees, her hair dragging on the floor,
now she can hear another woman outside, fiddling with
    the key, jiggling the lock & so she calls out Just a minute the
blood, she sees, tilting her face to the bowl, is crumbling out,
    bricks from a ruined fortress. Overhead, the fan's
dull rumble scatters dust like ashes & the tick
    as one blade catches each time it sweeps
past. One more wave & she crumples the paper in her hand
    wiping the sweat from her face, then wiping the blood. She
stands, ready to go back to where the men are discussing
    the scene with the baseball bat & the body
in the trunk of the Cadillac.

Esta Spalding

MRS. BARLOWE'S PLUM TREE

All summer the grass grows long
in the school yard across from Mrs. Barlowe's lawn

where the plums in the plum tree ripen

All summer I walk past to gauge
their purpling
until one August evening
their flesh is bruised as twilight
Plums heavy with their own
possibility

When Mrs. Barlowe sees me she
descends the steps from the porch

one hand on the rail
one hand on her cane

My son is coming to pick them
as soon as they ripen

Mrs. Barlowe nods to the school yard
past the chain link fence &
two empty soccer goals expectant
as two women

I'd offer them to you but my son
would be disappointed

She goes back up the steps closes
the door
I pick the plums for her

dropping them one by one
into the bucket

Tomorrow she'll tell me her son came

*

Actually there were crows on the branches
of the plum tree
purple-feathered in the twilight

The Sufis say the bird that flew
to look for paradise finally found it
in a mirror

These are not plums you'd put
in the fridge leaving a note to your lover
These plums taste like lemons
Evil plums Stepmother plums

Last time D went shopping
there were eight different kinds of pepper
on his list

Who needs eight different kinds of pepper?

The point is he does the shopping

There is no Mrs Barlowe

The Egyptian hieroglyph for mother

is the same as the one for death
a lappet-faced vulture

That tree belongs to no one
but the crows

& even they won't eat the plums

There is no plum tree
After I dreamt it
I cut it down

Esta Spalding

TRAIN WINDOW

Dawn on the train, my face
pressed against rocking

glass. Your head leaning on
my shoulder, hands in my lap, you

reach for sleep made difficult
by grief or love. Outside

bare birch. A glacial
river enunciates the cold.

Sometimes the nest of an eagle, but
never the eagle.

Raw sliver of sunlight breaks
between mountains. It pierces the window,

articulating a space between
our bodies.

After we lost the child, I picked up
the uncarved pumpkin &

cut it in half, raking fingers through the saffron
flesh, loosening the seeds.

I was going to salt & roast them, but
forgot, leaving them in a bowl on the counter

where they sprouted. A handful
of long shoots, expectant

lifting their shells on small green shoulders, craving
light. Each meal we prepared we

watched them, delirious with their own
growing, eating themselves

to stay alive. One morning they were
limp & straggly, draped over the lip

of the bowl, like mountain climbers who expire
in thin air, leaving their slumped bodies on the top

of the world.
The other day, stepping

out of the shower, mist around your
hips & shoulders, you let yourself

smile, *What are we going to do
with this love?*

The train stops. A freight's in trouble
further up the track & we are frozen

on steel spanning another river.
Ahead where the air is thinner

we cannot see. Behind
we can't turn back.

What are we going to do
with this love? Sun roses snow

on the branches. I lift my face from
the window glass.

We're tied to each other.
Where you climb, I will

climb. This light, ungraspable,
all we have.

Primus St. John

WATERING THE ORCHIDS

Sunlight at the window,
Another one of her brazen creatures
Pulling the eyes right out
Of the dark.
She and the shades are up,
Her cotton dress another blinding spectacle.
She imagining the luster of beings she whispers to,
Some of them tall, slim dancers, some gorgeous, lithe
Animals bouncing out of the blacksmith fire,
Some fickle divinities as unpredictable as birdsong.
She pouring her invocations to the day's verities
And I a sweet acolyte
With his grandmother in a forest of plants
And flowers at our living room window,
And now your grandfather,
Still pouring water for her.

Primus St. John

BATEY TUMBA

They are here along the road
Like bad teeth
Gnawing at miles and miles
Of luxurious cane.

Sometimes, I don't understand
Beauty at all,
Its art and devout community:
Twisted shacks
Bright paint
Dirt floors
And corrugated roofs
That are like feral animals

And its biblical story
Festered there for hundreds of years,
About little David's dark intuitive grace
And rhythmical confidence
That with a stone as small as this
You can go on.

Clemens Starck

NEIGHBORS

New neighbors
building a house up on the hill . . .
She raises goats. He works at the pen.
From my back door
it's thirty miles, as the crow flies,
over the mountains to the coast. It used to be
I could imagine
walking it—unimpeded.
No fences. Nothing but deer trails and logging roads.

Now I'm surrounded by neighbors.

Which is better: seeking the recluse
in the mountains, and finding he's not at home,
or helping the goat-lady
rig up a new wooden pedestal
for our mailboxes?

Clemens Starck

THE GIRL FROM PANAMA

I'm talking with Mike over coffee.
His wife recently left him. He's lonely.
We're both carpenters, a couple of old guys in baseball caps
plying the trade.
We can frame a wall and hang a door, we can
read a set of blueprints.
But when it comes to women . . .

I'm thinking about my mother, who is 91
and very frail. I'm thinking
about my wife, my daughters, my grand-daughter,
my sister, old girlfriends, my ex-wife,
and the girl from Panama
in the reading room of the New Orleans public library
forty-five years ago
who slipped a note to me across the table, asking:
"Are you a philosophy?"

Rain splatters against the storefront
of the coffee shop. Mike and I are silent
for a long time
before going back to work.

Lisa M. Steinman

GROGGINESS

Sometimes when you wake
your dreams hold on.

You drag them like ballast
through the day. Sleep tries

to repatriate you. As if
you won't move soon enough.

Your passport carries marks
of your commerce with the dead.

Lisa M. Steinman

HALTING MEDITATION

Everything grinds to a stop, which means
closed, but also *filled* up or *clogged*. Like *stuff*.
As in sated by the material

world. Or furnished. Full of substance. So
when one pulls out all the stops, nothing is
released, airy as music or thought.

Sandra Stone

ON THE BOULDERS OF INANITY

Every day terminates the clock—it, with
its driven tick, the orbit of numerals

peregrination of the hands (little
inexorables that encapsulate

air). I can't countenance math
its shoulder-less columns

sums like whirligigs—or
stats, their horrific rank

photos of dire embrace
the lostness of things

Statuesque, the women, marble-armed
lodge among besotted palms

anthem for planet's encoded data
set out like a table

From the balustrade, an overlook
I see the ocean's sated

Half-way across the world
vine-leaf's coppery stragglers

are at it again, boulders
like shrouded mourners

Compact Rodins
heads bent

Nothing is, that does not
cry out from its habitat

I hear the sound of brasses
Tinny for a coda

Drum roll of waves, inane music
in the migration of events

Joan Swift

LIGHT YEARS

Is light the last thing lost or never lost at all?
There is light so far away, it's gone

by the time we see it,
the tail lights on the highway far ahead

that say someone is travelling
this same dark way.

Those blue clumps lost ten billion light
years ago at the edge of the universe

redshift from ultraviolet to the visible
and are found by the Hubble telescope,

sleek horse pulling through dark
the reeling carriages of space

even as they change into roses
or thunderheads or phantom animals

we never imagined.
What fiery dust was our beginning,

left us a tender earth? Far out in the universe
a tomorrow we can't see is singing the last word

of a song we heard long ago under stars
like blossoms on black water.

Joan Swift

STEELHEAD

Because they flicker like stars of the twelfth magnitude
and have come all the way from the Bering Sea
through the Gulf of Alaska up the glacier-gray water
of the Copper River and then curved their backs to the plunge
of the Hanagita where they rest now, or have fallen
half conscious into this small green pool
fringed with spruces and scrub grass, you may think
they know something about endurance. Loneliness. Hope.
Or even birth and rebirth, their journey's reason.
When I stand with my shadow across the water
they are almost visible, finning in the place of my heart.
Then we bait our hooks and cast, lines floating out
toward the Wrangells, lures settling into the ripples
and riding downstream on a slant of September sunlight.
We do this one by one and one by one they wake up
to the transparent insect wing or the blackness
of raven down or the sweet round salmon egg.
They rise, are taken, and thrash—the bubbles silver,
the clouds of foam, hard runs over the gravel bottom.
All afternoon they are hooked and we let them go,
the same stunned fish over and over. We let them go.
Like all who desire and desire, they know nothing.

Mary Szybist

TOUCH GALLERY: JOAN OF ARC

> *The sculptures in this gallery have been carefully treated with a*
> *protective wax so that visitors may touch them.*
> *Exhibitions,* The Art Institute of Chicago

Stone soldier, it's okay now.
I've removed my rings, my watch, my bracelets.

I'm allowed, brave girl,
To touch you here, where the mail covers your throat,
Your full neck, down to your shoulders,
To here, where raised, unlatchable buckles
Mock fasten your plated armor.

Nothing peels from you.

Your skin gleams like the silver earrings
You do not wear.

Above you, museum windows gleam October.
Above you, high gold leaves flinch in the garden,

But the flat immovable leaves entwined in your hair to crown you
Go through what my fingers can't.
I want you to have a mind I can turn in my hands.

You have a smooth and upturned chin,
Cold cheeks, unbruisable eyes,
And hair as grooved as fig skin.

It's October, but it's not October
Behind your ears, which don't hint
Of dark birds moving overhead,
Or of the blush and canary leaves

Emptying themselves
in slow spasms
into shallow hedgerows.

Still bride of your own armor,
Bride of your own blind eyes,
This isn't an appeal.

If I could I would let your hair down
And make your ears disappear.

Your head at my shoulder, my fingers on your lips—

As if the cool of your stone curls were the cool
  Of an evening—
As if you were about to eat salt from my hands.

Mary Szybist

KNOCKING OR NOTHING

Knock me or not, the things of this world
Ring in me, shrill-gorged and shrewish

Clicking their charms and their chains and their spouts.
Let them. Let the fans whirr.

All your penitent virgins must have emptied
Their flimsy pockets, and I

Was empty enough,
Sugared and stretched and dazed on the un-mown lawn

Dumb as the frost-pink tongues
Of the un-pruned roses.

When you put your arms around me for that moment,
When you pulled me to you and leaned back,

When you lifted me just a few inches,
When you shook me

Hard then, had you ever heard
Such emptiness?

You knew I had room for every girl's locket,
Every last dime and pocketknife.

O my out-sung, fierce, unthinkable—
Why rattle only the world

You placed in me? Won't you clutter the unkissed,
Idiot stars? They blink and blink

Like quiet shepherds,
Like brides-about-your-neck.

Call them out of their quietness.
Knock them from nothing, from their empty enamel,

From the dark that has no way to hold them
And no appetite.

Call in the dead to touch them.
Let them slip on their own chinks of light.

Sharon Thesen

THE DAY LADY DI DIED

We'd spent the weekend at Bumbershoot
among the tents & booths of magick, then wound
back down apres the concluding events
past booths & tents deserted as Araby, down
to the Monorail station.

Lady Di, Lady Di, we heard up and down
the aisles—that's what they called her,
Lady Di. A car crash. It was
unbelievable. You're kidding, we said.

But there it was on the hotel room TV.
Solemn commentator, closed-off tunnel,
shots of wreckage. I started feeling homesick &
longed to hear her properly called Diana
Princess of Wales, watch her step
from a limousine wearing a moon-colored
evening gown, comfort patients at the hospice.

We didn't like being so far away from her style
& her death & hastened to the border
first thing in the morning.

Nance Van Winckel

YOU PEOPLE

People, don't ask me again where my shoes are.
The valley I walked through was frozen to me
as I was to it. My heavy hide, my zinc
talisman—I'm fine, people. Don't stare
at my feet. And don't flash the sign of the cross
in my face. I carry the Blue Cross Card—
card among cards, card of my number
and gold seal. So shall ye know I am of
the system, in the beast's belly and up
to here, people, with your pity.

People, what is wrong with you? I don't care
what the sign on your door says. I will go
to another door. I will knock and rattle
and if *you* won't, then surely someone, somewhere,
will put a pancake in my hand.

You people of the rhetorical *huh*? You lords and ladies
of the blooming stump, I bend over you, taste you,
keep an eye on you, dream for you the beginning
of what you may one day dream an end to.

The new century peeled me bone-bare
like a song inside a warbler—the bird
who knows not to go where the sky's stopped.
Keep this in mind. Do you think
the fox won't find your nest? That
the egg of you will endure the famine?

You, you people born of moons with no
mother-planets, you who are back-lit,
who have no fathers in heaven, hear now
the bruise-knuckled knock of me. I am returned.

From your alley. From your car up on blocks.
From the battered, graffitied railcars that uncouple
and move out into the studded green lightning.

Do you believe because your youth's
been ransacked, nothing more will be asked of you?
A bloody foot across your lawn?
Confuse me not with dawn. And people,

about the shoes: the shoes have no doubt entered the sea
and are by now walking the ramparts of Atlantis.
I may be a false prophet, but god bless me, at least
I have something to say. Supine in a pencil of night,
I've no chiseled tip yet, but already
the marks take form in the lead.

Nance Van Winckel

SIMONE WEIL AT THE RENAULT FACTORY (1935)

A thread in a line of threads, she stands
at the far end of her self. Eyelets and inlets,
divots for ingots. Migraines are the grain
of the day. In the awl's hollows, the nothing
God is to teach us the nothing we are.

The coupe is a cave. Go in and kneel
on its seat. Hands tool the tools
without us: to work to eat; to eat to work.

Where are the streets for such vehicles? Not yet
made. Where's the fuel to make go Go?
Underground, still pressing itself to become itself.

Punched-in lead holes; the head aches
when it's emptied out. A cold outside
comes in. The coupe is a cave.
Shine its horn; buff its blast.

The cave wheels forth—God,
where is it going? Into more rat-a-tat-
tat. More hands, less us; more air
in the airguns, less loud the heart.

Nance Van Winckel

UP THE STEPS OF THE CAPITOL

In line with many strangers,
we were roughed-up bodies
ready for more. We clasped hands.
A song made us iron. The line of us
could walk and sing. The line of us went on
and on—up the steps of the capitol and out
into towns with quarter-inch phonebooks.
Some in line knew the gods
and some their vices and others
how much was required of us
or just how rough it was
about to get. And the line of us
shrugged when we heard. We
were iron. From the purest
ore. This was after warnings
but before forbidding. Before
the dead came in waves, heavier
each time in our arms. Before
we had no hand free to close their eyes.
Still, for a while the rain seemed
nothing. We lashed ourselves
to ourselves. We were a line. Un-
crossable. The line of us could walk
and weep and believe we were of use.

Karen Volkman

SONNET

Sweetest bleeding is the cipher of sleep.
Soundless loaming, burying its dead.
The raw rilled lexicon that no one read.
No word survives the color of this deep,

this black unsinging—the wave escapes the leap,
its edges flatten—a syllable, a said
spell like pearl an ocean bore and bled
dying in harrows. Palliative, a sweep

blacks and satins. Sad sirens burn and sigh,
caressing the umber inner of a thigh—
unfolding in the flimmer of their hair

the swimming timbre, the wakeful stare
loosens its wooings, and wakes to die
drowning mutely, hollow as the sky.

Karen Volkman

SONNET

Bitter seed—scarred semblance—Psyche
sows the portion of contagion, liberty
in nerve and number, Cupid's quiddity
who catalogues the adage, zed to z,

and spends the nothing lovers' numbing plea
It shall be if we kiss it. Stone can see
what factors fault its fathoms, ardor we
mistake for fracture. A split, a volt, a v

of vain misgiving, void's elected be
knowing no rapture but its own redundancy.
So vowels do not die. They scale and scree

and haunt the planets with a harmony
as the zodiac wheels its pale menagerie
of soundless animals no love can free.

Karen Volkman

SONNET

Nothing was ever what it claimed to be,
the earth, blue egg, in its seeping shell
dispensing damage like a hollow hell
inchling weeping for a minor sea

ticking its tidelets, x and y and z.
The blue beneficence we call and spell
and call blue heaven, the whiteblue well
of constant waters, deepening a thee,

a thou and who, touching every what—
and in the or, a shudder in the cut—
and that you are, blue mirror, only stare

bluest blankness, whether in the where,
sheen that bleeds blue beauty we are taught
drowns and booms and vowels. I will not.

David Wagoner

WHAT THE STONES SAY

It isn't written in stone,
We say, meaning we'll change
Our minds, maybe, if others
Would just change theirs a little
On that slippery, unyielding ground
On the other side of the table.

Our fathers, long before us,
Before they thought up how
To make words permanent,
Before the alphabet,
Chiseled out pictographs
And dabbled in graffiti.

And archeologists tell us,
In chronological order,
These shapes were in their minds,
These shapes went down on stone:
First, solar discs, the sun
Hard at the heart of being.

Then labyrinths, the strange
Pathways to the gods.
Next, forms of rigid order,
Geometrical designs.
Then people facing one way
On their knees, praying together.

Weapons of war and the hunt—
Knives, crude spears, and arrows—
Came next, then houses and plots,
Ceremonies of cults,
Sketches of massacres,
And men mating with beasts.

David Wagoner

DESIRE

Flies are on the alert,
    Even when posing
To groom their busy wings
    Or clear some of those eyes,
So all frogs, because
    They have to, have to
Know exactly what
    The tips of their tongues
Should do to satisfy
    Their natural desire
For a fuller life and stomach
    And have all proved it
Through numberless generations
    Of choristers and swarms
Of good examples. Even if frogs
    Are punished with a spark
Or a slight touch of acid,
    They persist. They pay
The price and will keep on
    Snapping flies in spite
Of this new pain. Yet at last
    Even these slow learners
Master their desire. They try
    And try to forget. But no matter
What the curious minds
    In curious laboratories
Have devised, no frog on earth
    Or in water, from a spring
Peeper, its tadpole tail
    Only half gone,
To an old bullfrog
    Under a lily pad,
Can be the least bit
    Tempted or forced to take

A fly sitting still, showing
　　　No sign of leaving
Where it is to go somewhere
　　　Else or of moving even
The least important part
　　　Of itself to a new position.
All frogs would starve to death
　　　Among motionless flies.

David Wagoner

FOR AN OLD WOMAN AT THE GATE

Your permission slip has been stapled, decoded, stamped,
   And handed over to the authorities,
       Some of whom scan you now
And ask you to spread your arms, expecting you to fly
   All by yourself. One wants to see the insides
       Of your shoes, your good shoes,
As if you'd been complaining. Then he tries
   To ruin the heels. One snatches your purse and stands there
       Rummaging through it, right in front of you,
Thinking you won't remember what he looks like.
   He takes your book away and shakes it
       Upside down, losing your place again.
He wants to know if you've been given a gift
   By a stranger, which was so long ago,
       It's none of his business now, not even yours.
People are watching you, being kept back
   From the scene of this accident, worried, afraid
       They might be forced to testify. Your belongings
Have all been carried off somewhere without you
   To the end of an endless belt, to be disposed of
       Or given to the poor. A woman is smiling
Into your face, urging you to get moving
   Into the lobby of the wrong hotel
       With the heat turned off. She's giving you
A piece of plastic, one of those new keys
   That never work, yet you're supposed to work it
       On the right floor, in the right hallway,
In front of perfect strangers watching you,
   Expecting you to be perfect, in the right door
       Of the right room where you can't possibly sleep.

David Wagoner

THOREAU AND THE QUAGMIRE

His boots would sink there, down where they belonged:
   In the muddy water on the dead and the newly born
      Jumble of life. He wanted to know and feel
What hadn't come to light yet, what might be keeping
   Its darkness to itself in what the townsmen,
      Even his good neighbors, were calling *waste land*.
Among those hummocks and through the ponds between them,
   He touched in the open air and with both hands
      The roots, the sprouts and stems, the unfolding leaves
And spikelets and, with both his feet in the muck,
   Found where they began. He said their names
      Over and over to himself. But he hardly knew
What to do with those same hands and feet
   In the houses of strangers. They would search for each other
      Nervously at his knees or between them or forget
The way into pockets. His backward or forward feet
   Might lose their places, might stagger him
      On carpets or polished hardwood, might make him lurch
Off-balance, might seat him awkwardly
   In the quagmire of a chair, with a host and hostess
      Talking and listening. He would try his best
To pay his respects by meeting their painful price
   Of time and attention, hoping they might be as rich
      As purslane, target weed, or evergreen lambkill.

Emily Warn

APPALACHIAN MIDRASH

For no man shall see Me and live . . .
and my Face shall not be seen."
(Exodus 32:20)

Then who is it you saw,
or what, sweetening the air?
Not the single white cloud
behind a hill of bare elms,
not the cloud splattered on the river,
not the undulating trunks,
not the wind-broken blue,
but their blend, a current
flowing between mud banks,
your shutters locked open.

And she lifted up her eyes and she saw.

No leaves yet to stop light from hurtling through.
The creek carries it on its back.
The forest floor stares, starry eyed
with white violets and bluebells,
with blood root and bleeding heart.
No heat. No mosquitoes. Just a few gnats
warming up, sugaring the breeze.

To see is to contemplate a thing until it is understood.
(Moses Maimonides, *Guide for the Perplexed*)

The Appalachian spring is too much
when it gets going sweet gums, red bud, dogwoods
spatter winter goodbye with mauve smudges,
with lime-yellow simmerings, with white hot spots
rolling up the hills to fire the leafless trees.

When the day blows gently
and the shadows flee,
set out, my beloved . . .
for the hill of spices!
　　　　(Songs of Songs 2:17)

No trails signs until you arrive
at Thompson's Shelter just as rain
scatters campfire ash, flecks the creek,
a storm slowly beginning.

I had heard you with my ears
But now I see you with my eyes.
Therefore I recant and relent.
　　　　(Job 42:5–6)

To see not as a subject but as subject to seeing.
What do you see? Branches firing into a pool:
pop, pop, splash. White sparks. Rain flints.
To be always looking for You, eyes cast up
scanning the gray sky held in boney sycamores,
eyes cast down noting rain pocking the creek,
modulating its rush as you rush up the mountain
looking for your seventy faces.

See I set before you this day ticks and honey, choose honey.

Each second seventy drops of rain tip the creek;
the rain collects and falls from mountain bowl
to creek, from creek to creek to river, from river to river
to the wide open pupil of the sightless sea.

Who is watching the creek make its way
over moss, over slick granite slabs, over gravel?
you are watching the creek, you are watching the rain
rivet pools with quick white-hot jabs.

The seventy faces of God are seventy drops of rain
falling each second into the pool.
They are the river Dipper bobbing seventy times
on a boulder before sipping a beakful,
before bathing in the cold oxygen rush.
Each bow, each drop unveils what cannot be seen.

Each second rain pocks the creek, each pock
radiates a circle, a radian circle, a moon,
a *samech*, a silver bowl, a *yamulke*, an egg,
an *esrog*, a wedding ring, a pool.

Look into the pool until your eyes are its mirror.
Look until your hair is wet as leaves,
look until your bones are stiff as branches without leaves.
Look until you stop looking and see
rain pocks, ripples, sky splatter, your sighting
here then there moving downstream.

Emily Warn

KUF: MNEMONIC

ox
house
bridge
door
window
pillar
sword
gate
snake
hand
palm
spur
water
fish
circle
eyes
mouth
avatar
holiness
creation
desire
prophecy

1. (alef) Which word struck the first number out of the formless void?
2. (beit) Where do wind and light soap off together in the rain?
3. (gimel) How do you count from zero to one?
4. (dalet) Is there an instant between life and death?
5. (hei) Do the interior of clouds have moons and planets?
6. (vav) When your shovel scrapes the moonlight on the water, do you stop digging?
7. (zayin) How do coyotes, hunters and angels mark their principalities?

8.   (chet) how do you mingle persimmons and prayers?

9.   (tet) Why pour light into a cracked vessel?

10. (yud) Why illumine nothingness then withdraw?

20. (kaf) How does the present tense withstand the nearness of God?

30. (lamed) Who taught language to be sanctuary?

40. (mem) Why do church spires, radio antennaes, skyscrapers fish in air?

50. (nun) What is the Name for what has no measure?

60. (samech) Who is your dove, your perfect one?

70. (ayin) See, I have set before you this day ticks and honey.

80. (pei) Whoever writes down the Torah burns it.

90. (tzaddik) What does a framed pedigree puchase in a forest with no mushrooms?

100. (kuf) Does God lead or follow or reconnoiter?

200. (reish) To find the square root of holiness, totter around thieves.

300. (shin) Is the invisible light at the base of a candle flame a throne or a hovel?

400. (tav) See how the human being comes forth naked into this world and when she departs, goes away empty, as it is written.

Ingrid Wendt

MUKILTEO FERRY

After the long drive north, relentless
the traffic, relentless the heightened news of yet
another alert

after each car, each truck, has clanged
from dock to steel-plated deck and parked, and I get out
to stand at the stern—

light wind, clouds breaking,
and the quaking of tethered engines,
beyond this iron chain the dark water churning—

without warning, the cloak of a great
calm descends upon me, like
the very word

"upon"—the way
it slows the sentence down—
a measured word, hinged—the way

fish, in their inscrutable
expressions, hang
immobile, as though rooted

each to its own place—
and I enter again into the beneficence
of the world of water

whose rhythms will not be hurried
into whose covenant,
under the ancient composure of stars,

we pull anchor and begin to sail.

John Witte

Y

This night   and no other

this cold   this memory   this darkness beyond

the station   these stars   this crunching of boots

on the platform   this woman   holding a child

the distant whistle   the gate   clanging

the child   arching his back

making   with his mother   a Y

this gasping   and shunting   these words

and none other   this train   arriving

this big   sad animal

Carolyne Wright

AFTER WE RECEIVED THE NEWS OF THE 100-MILE WIND

Laramie to Cheyenne

We thought the first lines we sent out
would cover it—our stolen children
gathered into the apron of the wind—
but this gale chilled the farthest corners
of our meaning. Empty hopper cars

lifted lightly as balsa off the tracks
and our first warning—a warmth
with a threatening undercurrent to it—
was confirmed. All over town, children
were opening drawers, pulling jackets
from closets, hurrying down walks
as if to the bus stop. Fists burrowing

their pockets for the proper change,
they didn't notice how their parents' feet
were rooted to the porches, their hands
gnarling in the very act of waving *Wait!*
Come back! Across the prairies,

wind revved up its engines,
sucked in darkness like a fuel.
The children vanished
over the horizon. We drew our hands back,
the last in a genealogy of shadows.
Nothing we could have offered
would ever have been enough.

For my mother

Robert Wrigley

FOR ONE WHO PRAYS FOR ME

I do not wish to hurt her, who loves me
and who asks for me only every blossom and more,

but in fact, when I say God I mean the wind
and the clouds that are its angels;

I mean the sea and its enormous restraint,
all its fish and krill just the luster of a heavenly gown.

And while it is true there are days when I think
something more must be in the wind than air, still I believe

the afterlife is dirt, but sweet, and heaven's coming back
in the lewd, bewhiskered tongue of an iris.

Robert Wrigley

NEWS

There's a mountain and a hundred miles
between me and the jazz station, but sometimes
I can live with the static, a kind of extra-tempo
air-drum percussion, the dead singer's voice
tanged by smokes and too much gin. Some days,
all I want is no news, none of the time.

On the other hand, this afternoon it wasn't music
pulled me up, but what the field guide calls
the black-chinned hummingbird's "thin, excited chippering."
It had got itself trapped in the garage, and though
the big door was open, it stayed in the window
through which it could clearly see a world.

By the time I heard it, it was so exhausted
it let itself be cupped in my slow man's hands,
and emitted, as I closed it in, a single chip then silence.
At the edge of the woods I knelt and opened my hands.
Not even thumb-thick, its body pulsed with breath,
its wings spread across my palm, its eyelash legs

sprawled left and right, indecorously. I stroked it
as lightly as I could, as I might not my lover's breast
but the down made seemingly of air thereon, and twice.
Then it flew, a slow lilt into the distance. For a while,
even peace seemed possible, in the background
Billie Holiday singing "Strange Fruit."

Robert Wrigley

LETTER TO A YOUNG POET

In the biographies of Rilke, you get the feeling
you also get now and then in the poems
that here, surely, is a man among the archetypes of all men
you'd rather hang than have notice your daughter.
And yet, how not to admire the pure oceanic illogic
of his arguments, those preposterous
if irremediable verities. It can't be helped. They're true.
And there's no other word for him, for whom sadness is
a kind of foreplay, for whom seduction
is the by-product of the least practical art there is.
Those titanic skills in language, the knack lacked by
every other lung-driven swimmer through the waters
of lexicon, in spite of the fierce gravities of all grammar
and the sad, utilitarian wallflowers of usage:
well, there you go, my half-assed angel, that's your challenge.
Beethoven believed he was homely too, but you
must understand: Rilke's tools you can pick up, every one
but the one they all share. Even Stevens,
who must have known an actuary or two and still for whom
the brown salt skin of order sang beyond and in the ache
of longing. And Celan, whose most terrible angels
rang him like a bell of rings. And Whitman,
the dandy of the cocked hat and tilted head himself,
the gentlest, the gentile Jew, the jubilant lonely grubber
eyeing the grocery boy. Inside
them all, a man, if you could help it,
you would never consent to become,
except if only, just for once, you could be him.

Derk Wynand

KISSING BOOTH

she said in the kissing booth waiting
for the man who walked by to turn but
he did not turn and later denied it

the man later said kissing booth almost
as she had and described it for her
just the same in details all blue

as in persian she said blue as in baby blue
sky blue water and all of it more question
for him than even her kissing booth was

larks twittering in it sparrows on it and
their hearts all aflutter then those imported
starlings they'd shake their fists at what

did they know flying into and out of the blue
and he felt it later like a fist on the chest
the pressure hardest when he most denied it

and when he denied it again the kissing
booth his hair turned white and had he seen it
he would have denied that too and she

who did see said age makes no difference
but he knew the kissing booth had closed
the birds had startled up regrouped and

flown away and the silence after
was a harder proof than he would have chosen
for the birdlessness and the difference

Derk Wynand

REINED IN

Don't think *horse*, she said, but think of the thought
as one galloping away, then rein it in. Rein it in,

rein it in, she said, and return to the breath, yours or that
of the horse of which by now you should not be thinking.

Think of the reins, think of the bridle, think of white clouds
and scudding gowns. No, she said, think of the breath.

The thought still trotted toward a greener pasture. It fixed on
oats, fixed on alfalfa, and then on mare, though the mare

may have been human. Rein it in, she said. Just breathe
and focus on the breath. The breath entered, as it does,

by way of the nostrils, which flared at the very thought of it,
and the flaring led to other thoughts that had nothing much

to do with the breath, except they made his breathing
heavier. Rein it in, she said, and the air entered his lungs,

easier, and he held the thought there, held it, held
and expelled it. The mare still snuffled and snorted

in the green pasture and the thought could not help itself,
still wanting it human. Breathe, she said, and he did so.

Think of the breath, and he did, her eyes closed, her hands
placed just so in her lap, her chest just so also, rising, falling.

Her chest rose and fell and he steadied his thoughts,
focused them on the breathing and his breath stayed there.

Patricia Young

BUSTED

for singing in the school stairwell,
you and the Chinese grocer's
anorexic daughter. In the principal's office
she removed her stiff black hair
as though removing a hat.
It was Biology you'd escaped from,
the frog's heart and surgeon's tools.
How do we learn to forget,
she sang long ago in the school stairwell,
her bald head and unblinking eyes.
How indeed, the principal answered,
before sending you back
to your formaldehyde classroom.
Though for all you knew
the grocer's daughter
might have been asking,
What does death taste like?
She might have been singing to the trays
of tailless amphibians,
their brains washed in dying light.

⊞ BIOGRAPHIES OF THE POETS

JAN LEE ANDE

Jan Lee Ande was born in Tacoma, Washington. She comes from a long line of Anglican clergy, was in initiated into Tibetan Buddhism, and later joined a Roman Catholic community. Ande's poetry is influenced by the spiritual work of Rilke, Chagall, and Tantric art, and offers itself as a form of spiritual invocation. She lives in Portland.

Instructions for Walking on Water, Ashland Poetry Press, 2001
Reliquary, Texas Review Press, 2003

GINGER ANDREWS

The youngest of six children, Ginger Andrews was born in North Bend, Oregon, in 1956; her father was from Missouri and her mother from Arkansas. She wrote her first poem when she was ten years old, after her mother died. Andrews still lives in North Bend and works as a professional house cleaner. She has said that her poetry wants to fuse the crazy with the profound, something akin to scrubbing stains off a linoleum floor that obviously needs replacing.

An Honest Answer, Story Line Press, 1999
Hurricane Sisters, Story Line Press, 2004

JUDITH BARRINGTON

Judith Barrington was born in Brighton, England, in 1944, during the air raids of World War II. Both her parents drowned in a boating accident when she was nineteen, after which she lived in Spain for three years. These two events have influenced her work immensely. She moved to the Northwest in 1976 and is a naturalized U.S. citizen. Her poetry carries the imprint of her earliest literary influences: the British romantics, Adrienne Rich, Sylvia Plath, and Mimi Khalvati. She believes in the ideal that poetry is something that can be trusted as a source of wisdom.

Deviation, Women's Press, 1975
Trying to Be an Honest Woman, Eighth Mountain Press, 1985
History and Geography, Eighth Mountain Press, 1989
Horses and the Human Soul, Story Line Press, 2004

JOHN BARTON

The son of a Royal Air Force pilot, John Barton was born in Edmonton, Alberta, in 1957. He spent childhood summers in Victoria, B.C., and moved there in the late seventies to study writing at the University of Victoria. After a twenty-year hiatus from the Northwest when he worked in Ottawa for the Canada Aviation Museum, the National Gallery of Canada, and as co-editor of the journal *Arc*, he returned in 2004 to become the editor of *The Malahat Review*. His poems have long displayed a fascination with the moods of imagery as he explores the intersection between the private and the aesthetic.

A Poor Photographer, Sono Nis Press, 1981
Hidden Structure, Ekstasis Editions, 1984
West of Darkness: Emily Carr, a Self-portrait, Penumbra, 1987
Great Men, Quarry Press, 1990
Notes Toward a Family Tree, Quarry Press, 1993
Designs from the Interior, House of Anansi Press, 1994
Sweet Ellipsis, ECW Press, 1998
Hypothesis, House of Anansi Press, 2001
Asymmetries, Frog Hollow Press, 2004

BRUCE BEASLEY

Born in Thomaston, Georgia, in 1958, and raised in Macon, Georgia, with a twin brother and three older sisters, Bruce Beasley moved to Bellingham, Washington, in 1992 to teach at Western Washington University. His important influences are Emily Dickinson, Rainer

Maria Rilke, Theodore Roethke, Wallace Stevens, Gerard Manley Hopkins, and Charles Wright. Beasley sees poetry as a form of prayer and a place for emotional, spiritual, and linguistic extremity.

Spirituals, Wesleyan University Press, 1988
The Creation, Ohio State University Press, 1993
Summer Mystagogia, University of Colorado Press, 1996
Signs and Abominations, Wesleyan University Press, 2000
Lord Brain, University of Georgia Press, 2005
The Corpse Flower: New and Selected Poems,
    University of Washington Press, 2006

MARVIN BELL

Marvin Bell was born in 1937 in New York City and grew up on Long Island. His father emigrated as a teenager from Ukraine, and his mother was a first-generation American of Ukrainian parents. After serving in the Army during the mid-sixties, Bell had intended to settle in the Northwest, but in 1965 accepted a position teaching at the Iowa Writers' Workshop. He first came to the Northwest on the old Northwest Reading Circuit in the seventies and in 1985 bought a small house in Port Townsend, where he now lives most of the year. His earliest influences were the Beats, and his teachers—John Logan and especially Donald Justice—put him on the path toward writing poems, as he has said, that are "an expression of the otherwise inexpressible, an escape from time, and a message from the deep."

Things We Dreamt We Died For, The Stone Wall Press, 1966
A Probable Volume of Dreams, Atheneum, 1969
The Escape into You, Atheneum, 1971
Residue of Song, Atheneum, 1974
Stars Which See, Stars Which Do Not See, Atheneum, 1977
These Green-Going-to-Yellow, Atheneum, 1981
Segues: A Correspondence in Poetry (with William Stafford),
    David R. Godine, 1983
Drawn by Stones, by Earth, by Things That Have Been in the Fire,
    Atheneum, 1984
New and Selected Poems, Atheneum, 1987
Iris of Creation, Copper Canyon Press, 1990
A Marvin Bell Reader: Selected Poetry and Prose,
    University Press of New England, 1994
The Book of the Dead Man, Copper Canyon Press, 1994
Ardor: The Book of the Dead Man, Vol. 2, Copper Canyon Press, 1997

Wednesday: Selected Poems 1966–1997, Salmon Poetry, 1998
Poetry for a Midsummer's Night, Seventy Fourth St. Productions, 1998
Nightworks: Poems 1962–2000, Copper Canyon Press, 2000

JAMES BERTOLINO

Born in the Upper Peninsula of Michigan in 1942, James Bertolino grew up in a family of iron-ore miners. He lived in the Northwest briefly, in Eugene, in the late sixties, and later attended graduate school at Cornell. Afterward he taught at the University of Cincinnati. Bertolino's earliest influences began with the Beat poets—especially Gregory Corso and Allen Ginsberg, then segued to Gary Snyder, Robert Creeley, and Denise Levertov. In 1984 he moved to Washington State. His poems, he says, attempt to capture the peculiarities of humanity.

Employed, Ithaca House, 1972
Making Space for Our Living, Copper Canyon Press, 1974
The Gestures, Bonewhistle Press, Brown University, 1975
New and Selected Poems, Carnegie Mellon University Press, 1978
Precinct Kali & The Gertrude Spicer Story, New Rivers Press, 1982
First Credo, Quarterly Review of Literature, 1986
Snail River, Quarterly Review of Literature, 1995
Pocket Animals, Egress Studio Press, 2002

LINDA BIERDS

Linda Bierds was born in 1945 in Wilmington, Delaware, moved several years later to Anchorage, and later to Seattle, when her father, a pilot during World War II, took a position with Alaska Airlines. Her earliest influences include Elizabeth Bishop, James Dickey, James Wright, and Robert Bly, as well as the metaphor-drenched work of sixteenth- and seventeenth-century Dutch and Flemish painters. At the heart of Bierds's poetry is a concern with the mystery of phenomenon, rendered in exquisitely lyric monologues. She lives on Bainbridge Island.

Flights of the Harvest-Mare, Ahsahta Press, 1985
The Stillness, the Dancing, Henry Holt and Company, 1988
Heart and Perimeter, Henry Holt and Company, 1991
The Ghost Trio, Henry Holt and Company, 1994
The Profile Makers, Henry Holt and Company, 1997
The Seconds, Putnam, 2001
First Hand, Putnam, 2005

ANNE CASTON

Born in 1953 in Arkadelphia, Arkansas, first-born in a family of five children, Anne Caston was raised in a working-class, Southern Baptist community. Reading the Psalms, hymns, and stories of prophets had an early effect on her developing sense of poetry, and these experiences were reinforced by studying with Tom Sexton and Lucille Clifton. She came to Alaska the first time in the early eighties to work as a nurse. Working with patients on the graveyard shift, gravitating between what she has called "the lit world and the underworld," has given her work a blend of the scientific and the lyric. She returned to Alaska in 1999 and teaches in Anchorage at the University of Alaska.

Flying Out With The Wounded, New York University Press, 1997

KEVIN CRAFT

Kevin Craft was born in 1967 in Wilmington, Delaware. He has spent a good deal of time traveling, especially in the Mediterranean region, where he returns each year. In 1993 he moved to Seattle to complete an MFA at the University of Washington. Craft's earliest influences include James Wright, Seamus Heaney, and Wallace Stevens. He's attracted to sound in poetry, the materiality of the image, precision, and the metaphysical musing inherent in poetic expression—all as a process and act of discovery.

Solar Prominence, Cloud Bank Books, 2005

LORNA CROZIER

Born in 1948 in Swift Current, Saskatchewan, Lorna Crozier moved to the Northwest in 1991 to teach at the University of Victoria. Her father was a seasonal oil-field hand and her mother cleaned houses for grocery money. Her earliest interest in poetry was to preserve something of her parents' hard-scrabble life, to affirm that they mattered though the mark they made in the world, she has said, was small and erasable, except to their kin. For Crozier, poetry is the path to primal things, be they words, memory, or dream.

Inside Is the Sky, Thistledown Press, 1976
Crow's Black Joy, NeWest Press, 1979
Humans and Other Beasts, Turnstone Press, 1981
No Longer Two People (co-written with Patrick Lane),
    Turnstone Press, 1981
The Weather, Coteau Books, 1983

The Garden Going On Without Us, McClelland & Stewart, 1985
Angels of Flesh, Angels of Silence, McClelland and Stewart, 1988
Inventing the Hawk, McClelland and Stewart, 1992
Everything Arrives at the Light, McClelland and Stewart, 1995
A Saving Grace, McClelland and Stewart, 1997
What the Living Won't Let Go, McCelland and Stewart, 1999
The Apocrypha of Light, McClelland and Stewart, 2002
Bones in Their Wings, Hagios, 2003
Whetstone, McClelland and Stewart, 2005

OLENA KALYTIAK DAVIS
The daughter of Ukranian immigrants, Olena Kalytiak Davis was born in Detroit in 1963 and moved to Alaska in 1993. Her poems trash and rescue the confessional mode practically simultaneously, and they possess a riveting diction. She's attracted to words, she once said, the way some people are attracted to shoes. She lives in Anchorage.

And Her Soul Out Of Nothing, University of Wisconsin Press, 1997
shattered sonnets love cards and other off and back handed importunities,
    Bloomsbury/Tin House, 2003

MADELINE DEFREES
Daughter of an orphan mother and a father who was a bookkeeper, Madeline DeFrees was born in Ontario, Oregon, in 1919. After graduation from St. Mary's Academy in Portland, she entered the Sisters of the Holy Names of Jesus and Mary, where she was known for many years as Sister Mary Gilbert. Influenced early by the work of Emily Dickinson, E. A. Robinson, and Gerard Manley Hopkins, she was drawn to poetry because, as she has said, it can be the repository of the secret, a way of understanding experience and imposing an order on it.

From the Darkroom, Bobbs-Merrill, 1964
When Sky Lets Go, George Brazillier, 1978
Magpie on the Gallows, Copper Canyon Press, 1982
The Light Station on Tillamook Rock, Arrowood Books, 1990
Imaginary Ancestors, Broken Moon Press, 1990
Possible Sibyls, Lynx House Press, 1991
Blue Dusk: New and Selected Poems 1951–2001,
    Copper Canyon Press, 2001
Spectral Waves: New and Uncollected Poems,
    Copper Canyon Press, 2006

ALICE DERRY

Alice Derry was born in 1947 in Portland and grew up in Oregon, Washington, and Montana. After some years away from the region, she returned to the Northwest in 1980. Derry came relatively late to the writing of poetry, following deep reading in the work of the novelist William Faulkner, as well as in the poetry of John Keats, W. B. Yeats, Theodore Roethke, and the influential 1970s anthology, *The New Naked Poets*. She studied with Lisel Mueller, Tess Gallagher, and Ellen Bryant Voigt. Her poems dramatize the link between their home in language and their home in the world.

Stages of Twilight, Breitenbush, 1986
Clearwater, Blue Begonia Press, 1997
Strangers to Their Courage, Louisiana State University Press, 2001

CANDICE FAVILLA

Candice Favilla was born 1949 in Chico, California, and grew up on an almond farm where the men in her family climbed the trees and beat the branches with heavy mallets to harvest the almonds, and the women raked and piled them onto canvas sheets. Walt Whitman is an early influence as is the prose of W. S. Merwin. Favilla writes what she calls "presentational" poems, where the mind is at work in the process of making itself and the world of the poem. She has lived throughout the American West: California, Colorado, Wyoming, Texas, and now in Bandon, Oregon.

Cups, University of Georgia Press, 1992
Things That Ease Despair, Custom Words, 2005

TESS GALLAGHER

Tess Gallagher was born in Port Angeles, Washington, in 1943, and grew up in the logging camps there where both her parents worked. Her first important teacher was Theodore Roethke, and she later studied with David Wagoner and Mark Strand. Her influences are diverse: Marianne Moore, Federico Garcia Lorca, Chinese poetry, the painters Alfredo Arreguin and Morris Graves, Buddhist readings and personal practice, and her relationship and marriage to the late Raymond Carver. She has spent part of nearly every year since 1968 in Ireland, and Irish literature and art have nourished her sense of using language at its most fervent pitch and intensity, where poetry can change "experience into a revelation, an opening out, an acknowledgement of life's severities and beauties."

Instructions to the Double, Graywolf Press, 1976
Under Stars, Graywolf Press, 1978
Willingly, Graywolf Press, 1984
Amplitude: New and Selected Poems, Graywolf Press, 1987
Portable Kisses, Capra Press, 1992
Moon Crossing Bridge, Graywolf Press, 1992
My Black Horse: New and Selected Poems, Bloodaxe Books, 1995
Dear Ghosts, Graywolf Press, 2006

GARY GILDNER

Born in 1938 in northern Michigan, Gary Gildner grew up with the talent and aspiration to play professional baseball. When an injury derailed his plans, he studied comparative literature at Michigan State University. He has lived in the Clearwater Mountains of Idaho since 1993.

First Practice, University of Pittsburgh Press, 1969
Digging for Indians, University of Pittsburgh Press, 1971
Nails, University of Pittsburgh Press, 1975
The Runner, University of Pittsburgh Press, 1978
Blue Like the Heavens: New and Selected Poems,
    University of Pittsburgh Press 1984
Clackamas, Carnegie-Mellon University Press, 1991
The Bunker in the Parsley Fields, University of Iowa Press, 1997

MICHELE GLAZER

Michele Glazer is a native Oregonian. She lives in Portland. Her poems are a distilled mixture between memory, invention, and desire.

It Is Hard to Look at What We Came to Think We'd Come to See,
    University of Pittsburgh Press, 1997
Aggregate of Disturbances, University of Iowa Press, 2004

PATRICIA GOEDICKE

Born in Boston into an Irish Catholic family in 1931, Patricia Goedicke was brought up in Hanover, New Hampshire, where her father was the first resident psychiatrist at Dartmouth College. Goedicke was first drawn to poetry listening to Robert Frost's lectures at Middlebury College when she was a student there; she later studied briefly with W. H. Auden in New York. Goedicke believes that poems are, as she has said, "auguries of hope, sign and seal of a vast linguistic history whose roots nourish us all." After living in Mexico for twelve years, she arrived in Montana in 1981 as a Visiting Poet at the University of Montana—and remained on the faculty until her death in 2006.

Between Oceans, Harcourt, Brace & World, Inc., New York, 1968
For the Four Corners, Ithaca House, 1976
The Trail That Turns on Itself, Ithaca House, 1978
Crossing the Same River, University of Massachusetts Press, 1980
The King of Childhood, Confluence Press, 1984
The Wind of Our Going, Copper Canyon Press, 1985
The Tongues We Speak: New and Selected Poems,
   Milkweed Editions, 1989
Paul Bunyan's Bearskin, Milkweed Editions, 1991
Invisible Horses, Milkweed Editions, 1996
As Earth Begins to End, Copper Canyon Press, 2000

JAMES GRABILL

James Grabill was born in Ohio in 1949 to professional musicians—his mother a pianist and his father a one-time member of the Toledo Symphony. He moved to Portland during the seventies. Grabill has been influenced by the meditative extravagances of T. S. Eliot, Robert Bly, Theodore Roethke, and Galway Kinnell, as well as a love for little magazines, especially such idiosyncratic and prominent journals as *Field*, *kayak*, and *Poetry Northwest*. Grabill's poetry seeks to be a complex convergence of thinking, feeling, and intuiting.

One River, Momentum Press, 1975
Clouds Blowing Away, Seizure and Kayak Books, 1976
To Other Beings, Lynx House Press, 1981
Listening to the Leaves Form, Lynx House Press, 1998
An Indigo Scent after the Rain, Lynx House Press, 2003
Finding the Top of the Sky, Lost Horse Press, 2005
October Wind, Sage Hill Press, 2006

NEILE GRAHAM

Neile Graham was born in Winnipeg, Manitoba, in 1958, and has lived in the Northwest most of her life, currently in Seattle. Her earliest influences include Robert Bringhurst, W. S. Graham, and Jorie Graham, as well as the artist Emily Carr. Studying with Robin Skelton and Richard Hugo led her to see poetry, as she has said, as "that spiral at the centre of the smallest part of us that describes who we are, our history, what that has made us and what we can make of it, describing both our ancestry, our present conditions, and the possibilities of our future."

Seven Robins, Penumbra Press, 1984
Spells for Clear Vision, Brick Books, 1994
Blood Memory, Buschek Books, 2000

CATHERINE GREENWOOD

The daughter of Scottish immigrants, Catherine Greenwood grew up on a cattle ranch on the international border in British Columbia's Boundary District and has lived most of her life on Vancouver Island. During her twenties, she abandoned writing, but returned to poetry when she undertook study with Lorna Crozier and Derk Wynand at the University of Victoria. Her poems display a fascination with the imagery of borderlines and identity.

The Pearl King and Other Poems, Brick Books, 2004

JOHN HAINES

John Haines was born in Norfolk, Virginia, in 1924, the son of a career Naval officer. During his childhood, he lived in Bremerton, Washington, where his father was stationed. He studied drawing and sculpture at American University after World War II and began writing poems during the first winter he homesteaded south of Fairbanks, Alaska. For Haines, poetry is a calling, not a profession, and a search for truth—as perceived in the shape and cadences of a poem.

Winter News, Wesleyan University Press, 1966
The Stone Harp, Wesleyan University Press, 1971
News from the Glacier: Selected Poems, Wesleyan University Press, 1983
New Poems, Story Line Press, 1990
The Owl in the Mask of the Dreamer: Collected Poems,
    Graywolf Press, 1993
At the End of This Summer, Copper Canyon Press, 1997
For the Century's End, Poems 1990–1999,
    University of Washington Press, 2001

KATHLEEN HALME III

Kathleen Halme III was born in the mining and logging regions of Michigan's Upper Peninsula in 1955. Her father was a meat cutter, her mother a nurse. Her early interest in anthropology and ethnography—as well as deep reading in the work of Charles Baudelaire, Wallace

Stevens, Emily Dickinson, and Alice Fulton—continue to influence her poems, which draw a reader's attention to an adroit sense of language and the roots of consciousness. She moved to Portland in 1997.

Every Substance Clothed, University of Georgia Press, 1995
Equipoise, Sarabande Books, 1998
Drift and Pulse, Carnegie Mellon University Press, 2006

SAM HAMILL

Sam Hamill was born in 1943 and was adopted at the age of three by a Utah farm family. At fifteen, he left home, and was in and out of jails before serving in the U.S. Marine Corp. He came to his life in poetry first under the influence of the Beats in the late fifties, and later thrived under the tutelage of Kenneth Rexroth. But Hamill's influences are broad: Ezra Pound, Tu Fu, Mississippi Delta blues, four decades practicing Zen Buddhism, political activism, and work as a prolific translator and essayist. For thirty-two years he was editor at Copper Canyon Press and has lived in and near Port Townsend, Washington, since 1974.

Petroglyphs, Three Rivers Press, 1975
The Calling Across Forever, Copper Canyon Press, 1976
Triada, Copper Canyon Press, 1978
Animae, Copper Canyon Press, 1980
Fatal Pleasure, Breitenbush Books, 1984
The Nootka Rose, Breitenbush Books, 1988
Mandala, Milkweed Press, 1992
Destination Zero: Poems 1970–1995, White Pine Press, 1995
Gratitude, BOA Editions, 2000
Dumb Luck, BOA Editions, 2003
Almost Paradise: New & Selected Poems & Translations, Shambhala, 2005

JERRY HARP

Jerry Harp grew up in Southern Indiana. His earliest influences include John Donne, William Cullen Bryant, Carl Sandburg, and T. S. Eliot. He moved to Portland, Oregon, to teach at Lewis and Clark College in 2004.

Creature, Salt Publishing, 2003
Gatherings, Ashland Poetry Press, 2004
Urban Flowers, Concrete Plains, Salt Publishing, 2006

JANA HARRIS

Jana Harris was born south of San Francisco and moved with her family to the holly farms and filbert orchards of the Clackamas River in Oregon when she was fifteen. She attended the University of Oregon and later San Francisco State University where she studied with Robert Creeley, Philip Lamantia, and Kay Boyle. She was a founder of *Poetry Flash* in Berkeley, director of the Manhattan Theatre Club's literary series, and editor and founder of *Switched-on Guttenberg*, one of the first on-line poetry journals. She lives in Washington. Her poems are re-imaginations of pioneer narratives.

The Clackamas, The Smith, 1980
Manhattan as a Second Language, Harper & Row, 1982
The Sourlands, Ontario Review Press, 1989
Oh How Can I Keep on Singing? Voices of Pioneer Women,
    Ontario Review Press, 1993
The Dust of Everyday Life, an Epic Poem of the Pacific Northwest,
    Sasquatch, 1997
We Never Speak of It, Idaho–Wyoming Poems, 1889–90,
    Ontario Review Press, 2003

GARRETT HONGO

Garrett Hongo was born in 1951 in the village of Volcano on the island of Hawai'i in the back room of his grandfather's general store. He grew up in O'ahu and later, as a teenager, in Los Angeles. He studied at Pomona College and lived in Japan. Hongo's earliest literary influence came from reading poetry in translation—Pablo Neruda, Miguel Hernandez, Yannis Ritsos, T'ang Dynasty poets—as well as from mentors such as Charles Wright, C. K. Williams, and the playwright Wakako Yamauchi. Hongo has called poetry "the most civilized part of being.

Yellow Light, Wesleyan University Press, 1982
The River of Heaven, Knopf, 1988

CHRISTOPHER HOWELL

Christopher Howell was born in Portland and grew up on his family's ancestral farm that the city has since overtaken. He began writing poems as a student at Pacific Lutheran University in Tacoma and later served as a Navy journalist during the Vietnam War. Howell studied with Henry Carlile, James Tate, Maxine Kumin, and Joseph Langland, and he immersed himself in the Deep Image poetry of W. S. Merwin,

Galway Kinnell, Robert Bly, and James Wright. His poetry is a means of reconciling the everyday world with the inner life, and he has said he hopes it acts as a "humane and primary response" to living. He lives in Spokane, Washington.

The Crime of Luck, Panache Books, 1977
Why Shouldn't I, L'Epervier Press, 1978
Though Silence: The Ling Wei Texts, L'Epervier Press, 1981
Sea Change, L'Epervier Press, 1985
Memory and Heaven, Eastern Washington University Press, 1996
Sweet Afton, True Directions, 1996
Just Waking, Lost Horse Press, 2003
Light's Ladder, University of Washington Press, 2004

HENRY HUGHES

Born in Port Jefferson, New York, in 1965, Henry Hughes grew up in two worlds: fishing and hunting along the sound, bays, and marshes of Long Island and spending time in the museums, libraries, strip joints, and bars of New York City. He lived for five years in Japan and China. Hughes is attracted to poetic narrative—"stories told in the mind's music," as he puts it, and his writing sets him in the company of the best of his own influences: James Dickey, Mary Oliver, Jack Gilbert, and his teacher, Li-Young Lee. Hughes moved to Oregon in 2002 and teaches at Western Oregon University.

Men Holding Eggs, Mammoth Books, 2004

LAWSON FUSAO INADA

A third-generation Japanese American, Lawson Fusao Inada was born in Fresno, California, in 1938. In 1942 his family joined other Japanese Americans in internment camps where they were confined for the duration of World War II. He was first incarcerated at the Fresno County Fairgrounds, then moved to a camp in Arkansas, and finally interned at a camp in Colorado at the end of the war. Inada was deeply influenced by jazz (he studied string bass). But as a student at Fresno State, he began writing poetry under the tutelage of Philip Levine. Inada's poetry addresses the multi-cultural flux of American life. He lives in Medford, Oregon.

Before the War: Poems as They Happened, Morrow, 1971
Legends from Camp, Coffee House Press, 1983
drawing the line, Coffee House Press, 1997

LAURA JENSEN

Born in 1948, Laura Jensen has lived in Tacoma, Washington, nearly her entire life. Her work has often centered on the most telling details of perception, as if what's seen has its own genealogy. Genealogy is an ongoing concern of hers, with projects that include translating song lyrics from Swedish and transcribing the life stories of her Danish, Swedish, and Finnish parents and grandparents.

Bad Boats, Ecco Press, 1977
Memory, Ecco Press, 1982
Shelter, Dragon Gate Press, 1985

JONATHAN JOHNSON

Jonathan Johnson was born in Fresno, California, and spent summers on a family ranch in Idaho, where he has lived off and on since 1996. His parents were deeply invested in literary life: his mother a scholar of the Romantics, his father a fiction writer. That, plus early reading of Jim Harrison and Galway Kinnell, steered his life toward poetry. His work records the fluid, cyclical relationship between imaginative and physical landscapes.

Mastadon, 80% Complete, Carnegie Mellon University Press, 2001
In the Land We Imagined Ourselves, Carnegie Mellon University Press, 2007

ARLITIA JONES

Arlitia Jones was born in 1965 in Pasco, Washington, and moved in 1971 to Anchorage, where her father worked as a butcher during the building of the Alaska pipeline. She studied with Tom Sexton and Linda McCarriston and today works in her family's wholesale meat shop, where she sometimes begins poems on the back of a calculator tape. Jones values freshness and accessibility in poetry.

The Bandsaw Riots, Bear Star Press, 2001

EVE JOSEPH

Born in North Vancouver in 1953, Eve Joseph worked for a time on freighters and has drawn on that experience at sea for her writing. Her influences are diverse: Yehuda Amichai and W. B. Yeats, Jane Kenyon and Ted Hughes, Pablo Neruda and Paul Celan. For many years she has worked with the dying at a hospice, and has sought to make, as she has said, a poetry that enters the darkness but asks nothing of it.

The Startled Heart, Oolichan Press, 2004

RICHARD KENNEY

Richard Kenney was born in Glens Falls, New York, in 1948, and moved to Seattle in 1984. Influenced early by the poetry of W. B.Yeats, W. H. Auden, Robert Frost, and James Merrill, Kenney's work is concerned with human evolution and the origins of language, as well as the cognitive basis of poetic forms. He lives in Port Townsend.

The Evolution of the Flightless Bird, Yale University Press, 1984
Orrery, Atheneum, 1985
The Invention of the Zero, Knopf, 1993

MICHAEL KENYON

Born in 1953 in Sale, Cheshire, England, Kenyon moved to Vancouver, British Columbia, when he was fourteen. Influenced by the poetry of Lawrence Ferlinghetti and the Beats, the music of Miles Davis, and the films of Wim Wenders, Werner Herzog, and Akira Kurosawa, Kenyon entered the writing of poetry, he has said, as if entering a sanctuary where he could map the altered states of his desires. His poems are a means to address the edges and transitions of both identity and relationships.

Rack of Lamb, Brick Books, 1991
The Sutler, Brick Books, 2005

JOANNA KLINK

Joanna Klink was born in Iowa City, Iowa in, 1969, and studied at Johns Hopkins and the University of Iowa. She moved to Missoula in 2000 to teach at the University of Montana. She is an ardent admirer of European poetry, especially the poems of Paul Celan, and her writing mixes quiet tones with intense emotional insight.

They Are Sleeping, University of Georgia Press, 2000

PATRICK LANE

Born in 1939 in Nelson, British Columbia, Patrick Lane had no formal education beyond high school. He first had his poetry published while he was working as a logger in northern British Columbia. He worked a variety of jobs, including truck driver, Cat skinner, chokerman, boxcar loader, industrial first-aid man, and as a clerk at a number of sawmills. Lane was active in the Vancouver poetry revival of the sixties. His poetry often deals with humanity's harshness and violence. He lives near Victoria.

Letters From the Savage Mind, Very Stone House, 1966
Separations, New Books, 1969

Mountain Oysters, Very Stone House, 1971
The Sun Has Begun to Eat the Mountain, Ingluvin Publications, 1972
Beware the Months of Fire, House of Anansi Press, 1974
Unborn Things: South American Poems, Harbour, 1975
Albino Pheasants, Harbour, 1977
Poems, New & Selected, Oxford University Press, 1978
The Measure, Black Moss Press, 1980
A Linen Crow, a Caftan Magpie, Thistledown Press, 1984
Selected Poems, Oxford University Press, 1987
Milford and Me, Coteau Books, 1989
Winter, Coteau Books, 1990
Mortal Remains, Exile Editions, 1991
Too Spare, Too Fierce, Harbour, 1995
Go Leaving Strange, Harbour, 2004

DORIANNE LAUX

Dorianne Laux was born in Augusta, Maine, in 1952, of Irish, French, and Algonquin heritage. She was raised in San Diego, California, spent a few years in West L.A., and in 1982 moved to Berkeley, where she lived for ten years. In 1992 she moved to Petaluma, California, and worked a variety of jobs, taught private poetry workshops, and published two books of poems before she began teaching at the University of Oregon in 1994. Laux's poetry seeks out the luminous in the ordinary and celebrates the possibilities of desire. She lives in Eugene.

Awake, BOA Editions, 1990
What We Carry, BOA Editions, 1994
Smoke, BOA Editions, 2000
Facts about the Moon, W.W. Norton, 2005

URSULA K. LE GUIN

Born in 1929, Ursula K. Le Guin grew up in Berkeley and the Napa Valley and has lived for over forty years in Portland. Though she is spoken of as a writer of science fiction and fantasy, the landscape of much of her fiction and most of her poetry is California and Oregon. She is best known as a novelist, but published poems before she published fiction, and continues both to write and translate poetry.

Wild Angels, Capra, 1974
Hard Words, Harper & Row, 1981
Wild Oats and Fireweed, Harper & Row, 1988
Going Out with Peacocks, HarperCollins, 1994

Sixty Odd, Shambhala, 1999
Incredible Good Fortune, Shambala, 2006

TOD MARSHALL

Born in 1967 in Buffalo, New York, Tod Marshall moved to the Northwest in his early twenties. He has studied with Nance Van Winckel and Daryl Murphy and was drawn early on to the poetry of Jack Gilbert and Hart Crane. An interest in the music and clarity of the lyric is of primary concern in his work.

Dare Say, University of Georgia Press, 2002

LINDA MCCARRISTON

Linda McCarriston was born in Chelsea Naval Hospital in Massachusetts during World War II and grew up in Lynn, Massachusetts. With few books at home, she discovered the neighborhood Bookmobile and local libraries and later read Henry Longfellow, W.B. Yeats, Edna St. Vincent Millay and e.e. cummings. Drawn to poetry as language with a fever, a rapid pulse, a great thirst, McCarriston sees poetry's social function as ancient, anarchic, and dangerous to power. She moved to Alaska in 1994 and lives in Fairbanks.

Talking Soft Dutch, Texas Tech University Press, 1984
Eva-Mary, TriQuaterly Books, Northwestern University Press, 1991
Little River, TriQuarterly Books, Northwestern University Press, 2002

FRANCES MCCUE

Frances McCue's childhood was spent in Ohio, Pennsylvania, and Massachusetts, where she was raised by her maternal grandparents and then by her mother and stepfather. Influenced by Richard Hugo, she has said she wants her poetry to rebel against the structures and puritanical traditions of the East Coast, as she sees it, in favor of the aesthetic expanses of the West Coast, where she has lived now for some twenty years.

The Stenographer's Breakfast, Beacon Press, 1992

ROBERT MCDOWELL

Born in 1953 in Alhambra, California, Robert McDowell moved to a seed and sheep farm in Browsnville, Oregon, in 1989. His influences are diverse: Lord Byron, Percy Shelley, Robinson Jeffers, Mickey Spillane, Isac Dinesen, and comic books; he studied with Raymond Carver,

William Jay Smith, and Mark Strand. McDowell's wide experience—as a newspaper columnist, farmer, traveler, tanner, housepainter, literary editor, baseball manager—have been included in his conception of poetry as a part of his spiritual practice, a way of communicating in the clearest possible way, and a way of carrying on the most important ongoing conversation given us, one's conversation with one's self.

Quiet Money, Henry Holt, 1987
The Diviners, Peterloo Poets, 1995
On Foot, In Flames, University of Pittsburgh Press, 2002

COLLEEN J. MCELROY

Colleen J. McElroy was born in St. Louis, Missouri, and traveled as a young woman in Europe and Mexico. In the mid-sixties, she moved to Bellingham, Washington, with her two children, and became an active presence in the Northwest's growing art and literary scene. Reading Richard Hugo, Gwendolyn Brooks, Al Young, and Anne Sexton informed her earliest work. Her poetry, she has said, strives to use all the senses to apprehend the physical.

Music From Home: Selected Poems,
    Southern Illinois University Press, 1976
Queen of the Ebony Isles, Wesleyan University Press, 1984
Bone Flames, Wesleyan University Press, 1987
What Madness Brought Me Here: New and Selected Poems,
    Wesleyan University Press, 1990
Travelling Music, Story Line Press, 1999

HEATHER MCHUGH

Heather McHugh was born to Canadian parents in San Diego in 1948. She was raised in Virginia and educated at Harvard University, where she studied with Robert Lowell. She moved to the Northwest in the early eighties to teach at the University of Washington. "My whole work is to catch the word by surprise, sneaking up on language, sneaking up on the world as it lurks in words," she has said, adding, "I love the recesses of reason." McHugh lives in Seattle.

Dangers, Houghton Mifflin, 1977
A World of Difference, Houghton Mifflin, 1981
To the Quick, Wesleyan University Press, 1987
Shades, Wesleyan University Press, 1988
Hinge & Sign: Poems 1968–1993, Wesleyan University Press, 1994

The Father of the Predicaments, Wesleyan University Press, 1999
Eyeshot, Wesleyan University Press, 2004

DON MCKAY

Don McKay was born in Owen Sound, Ontario, in 1942, and has lived in many Canadian provinces. His early efforts as a poet were influenced by the work of Ted Hughes, Sylvia Plath, and Al Purdy. For McKay, poetry is the place where language realizes its own inadequacy and, in a new condition of humility, speaks.

Sanding Down This Rocking Chair on a Windy Night,
   McClelland and Stewart, 1981
Birding, or Desire, McClelland and Stewart, 1983
Night Field, McClelland and Stewart, 1991
Apparatus, McClelland and Stewart, 1997
Another Gravity, McClelland and Stewart, 2000
Camber: Selected Poems 1983–2000, McClelland and Stewart, 2004
Strike/Slip, McClelland and Stewart, 2006

GEORGE MCWHIRTER

George McWhirter was born in Belfast, Northern Ireland, in 1939. At Queen's University Belfast, he studied with Laurence Lerner and was a classmate of Seamus Deane, Seamus Heaney, and Robert Dunbar. He taught in Kilkeel and Bangor, County Down, then in Barcelona, before coming to Port Alberni on Vancouver Island. From there, in the late sixties, he went to the University of British Columbia's Creative Writing Program and studied with J. Michael Yates. McWhirter taught at UBC until 2005. His poetry strives to make sense out of the senses, and as he says, to "sing with the synergy of the senses."

Catalan Poems, Oberon Press, 1971
Queen of the Sea, Oberon Press, 1976
Twenty Five, Fiddlehead Press, 1978
The Island Man, Oberon Press, 1981
Fire Before Dark, Oberon Press, 1983
A Staircase for All Souls, Oolichan Books, 1993
Incubus: The Dark Side of the Light, Oberon Press, 1995
The Book of Contradictions, Oolichan Books, 2002

JOSEPH MILLAR

Born in 1945 in Madison, Wisconsin, where his father was in the U.S. Army, Joseph Millar grew up in western Pennsylvania and Gloucester, Massachusetts. He moved to San Francisco in 1967 and Eugene in 1997. An important influence on Millar's imagination is popular music: Lightning Hopkins, Jimmy Reed, the Shirelles, Curtis Mayfield, Elvis Presley. He has long been attracted to poetry's secret side, the mysterious song of its language, as it attempts to speak something that can't be spoken.

Overtime, Eastern Washington University Press, 2001
Fortune, Eastern Washington University Press, 2006

SUSAN MUSGRAVE

Born in 1951 in Santa Cruz, California, Susan Musgrave was raised in British Columbia. She has spent extended periods of time living in Ireland, England, the Queen Charlotte Islands, Panama, and Colombia. Her poems have a deft habit of mixing tones: comedy with anger, tragedy with camp. She lives on Vancouver Island and on Haida Gwaii/Queen Charlotte Islands.

Songs of the Sea-Witch, Sono Nis Press, 1970
Entrance of the Celebrant, Macmillan, 1972
Grave-Dirt and Selected Strawberries, Macmillan, 1973
The Impstone, McClelland and Stewart, 1976
Selected Strawberries and Other Poems, Sono Nis Press, 1977
Becky Swan's Book, Porcupine's Quill, 1978
A Man to Marry, a Man to Bury, McClelland and Stewart, 1979
Tarts and Muggers: Poems New and Selected, McClelland and Stewart, 1982
Cocktails at the Mausoleum, McClelland and Stewart, 1985
The Embalmer's Art: Poems New and Selected, Exile Editions, 1991
Forcing the Narcissus, McClelland and Stewart, 1994
Things That Keep and Do Not Change, McClelland and Stewart, 1999
What the Small Day Cannot Hold: Collected Poems 1975–1980, Beach Holme, 2000

P. K. PAGE

P. K. Page was born in 1916 in Swanage, Dorset, England, and moved to Canada in 1919. She attended schools in Winnipeg, Calgary, and England, and studied at the Art Students' League and Pratt Graphics in New York. She worked as a sales clerk and a radio actress and edited several periodicals. Her work is full of inventive recoveries with a clear sense of memory as her conduit of the imagination. She lives in British Columbia.

Unit of 5, Ryerson, 1944
As Ten As Twenty, Ryerson, 1946
The Metal and the Flower, McClelland and Stewart, 1954
Cry Ararat! Poems New and Selected, McClelland and Stewart, 1967
Poems (1942–1973) Selected and New, House of Anansi Press, 1974
Evening Dance of the Grey Flies, Oxford University Press, 1981
The Glass Air, Oxford University Press, 1985
The Glass Air: Poems Selected and New, Oxford University Press, 1991
Hologram: A Book of Glosas, Brick Books, 1994
The Hidden Room: Collected Poems Volumes 1 & 2,
    The Porcupine's Quill, 1997
Alphabetical, Cosmologies, Poppy Press, 2001
Planet Earth, The Porcupine's Quill, 2002
Cosmologies, David R. Godine, 2003
Hand-Luggage: A Memoir in Verse, The Porcupine's Quill, 2006

SUZANNE PAOLA
Born in 1956 in Atlanta, Georgia, Suzanne Paola grew up in Elizabeth, New Jersey. Paola's poems honor the work of her earliest influences: Wallace Stevens, Sylvia Plath, Virginia Woolf, Charles Wright, and T. S. Eliot. Like her influences, her poems, too, are a form of serious play. Paola moved to the Northwest in 1992 and lives in Bellingham, Washington.

Petitioner, Owl Creek Press, 1986
Glass, Quarterly Review of Literature, 1995
Bardo, University of Wisconsin Press, 1998
The Lives of the Saints, University of Washington Press, 2002

GREG PAPE
Greg Pape was born in Eureka, California and studied at Fresno State University with Philip Levine, Peter Everwine, Charles Hanzlicek, and Robert Mezey. He has been an itinerant teacher at Hollins College, University of Missouri-Columbia, University of Alabama, and University of Louisville, among others. In 1987 he began teaching at the University of Montana where he worked alongside and became deeply influenced by Richard Hugo. Pape's poems are a means of concentration and paying attention to the world & one's life in the world.

Border Crossings, University of Pittsburgh Press, 1978

Black Branches, University of Pittsburgh Press, 1984
Storm Pattern, University of Pittsburgh Press, 1992
Sunflower Facing the Sun, University of Iowa Press, 1992

MIRANDA PEARSON

Miranda Pearson spent the first thirty years of her life in England. She began writing poetry after she moved to Vancouver, Canada. She received an MFA in creative writing from the University of British Columbia, and now works as the poetry "mentor" at Simon Fraser University's Writer's Studio. Her poems are investigations of displacement and artifice.

Prime, Beach Holme, 2001
The Aviary, Oolichan Press, 2006

PETER PEREIRA

One of ten children, Peter Pereira was born in Spokane in 1959. He attended the University of Washington as an undergraduate. After taking degrees in English and Biology, he went to medical school and now practices in West Seattle. His most important early reading includes the work of Frank O'Hara, Carolyn Forché, Louise Glück, and Charles Wright. Interested in a casual style, Pereira sees poetry as means to hold experiences to the light, to understand them, and to heal or grow from them.

Saying the World, Copper Canyon, 2003

LUCIA PERILLO

Lucia Perillo grew up in the suburbs of New York City in the 1960s and attended college outside of Montreal, where she majored in Wildlife Management. When she graduated, she lived for a brief period on a commune run by women and began working for the U.S. Fish and Wildlife Service in Denver. While working at a wildlife refuge in San Francisco, she studied with Robert Hass, and later with Philip Booth, Hayden Carruth, Stephen Dobyns, and Tess Gallagher. Perillo first came to Washington state in 1988 to be a ranger at Mount Rainier and during this time learned that she had multiple sclerosis. She lives in Olympia.

Dangerous Life, Northeastern University Press, 1989
The Body Mutinies, Purdue University Press, 1996
The Oldest Map with the Name America, Random House, 1999
Luck is Luck, Random House, 2005

PAULANN PETERSEN

Paulann Petersen was born in 1942 in Portland, Oregon. Her father was a sheet-metal mechanic and her mother a nurse. Her influences are diverse: Rumi, Lucille Clifton, and William Stafford. Petersen has been a dedicated student of the art of poetry, taking classes from many poets, including Denise Levertov, Adrienne Rich, Carolyn Kizer, and Grace Paley. Her work dwells in the mysteries, silences, and capacities of the human heart—the heartbeat and breath of humanity. She has lived in Oregon her entire life.

The Wild Awake, Confluence Press 2002
Blood Silk, Quiet Lion Press, 2004
A Bride of Narrow Escape, Cloudbank Books, 2006

STEVEN PRICE

Steven Price was born in 1976 in Colwood, British Columbia. Besides a year in New Zealand and two years in Virginia, where he studied with Charles Wright, he has lived in British Columbia his entire life. His first influences include Seamus Heaney, Czeslaw Milosz, and Jack Gilbert— poets, like Price, who use memory to unearth the sources of experience and language.

Anatomy of Keys, Brick Books, 2006

JAROLD RAMSEY

Born in Bend, Oregon, in 1937, Ramsey was raised on a wheat and cattle ranch north of Madras. His parents were both children of homesteaders. Ramsey was drawn to poetry as an undergraduate at the University of Washington. William Stafford, Theodore Roethke, and W. S. Merwin were early influences on his work, as were American Indian stories and songs. His poetry has long been about celebration and conservation— celebrating living and conserving what life richly gives and takes away.

The Space Between Us, Adam Books, 1970
Love in an Earthquake, University of Washington Press, 1973
Demographia, Cornstalk Press, 1983
Hand-Shadows, Quarterly Review Press, 1989

CARLOS REYES

Born during the Depression in Southwest Missouri, Carlos Reyes came to Oregon during the forties. By 1953, he'd left the U.S. to travel and live in Panama. Reyes began writing poetry during the sixties while a student at the University of Arizona, influenced by Gary Snyder, Charles Olson, and especially Robert Creeley. His writing is plain-spoken and earnest and expresses a fascination with ecstatic occasions.

The Shingle Weaver's Journal, Lynx House, 1980
Nightmarks, Lynx House, 1990
A Suitcase Full of Crows, Bluestem, 1995
At the Edge of the Western Wave, Lost Horse Press, 2004

KATRINA ROBERTS

Katrina Roberts was born in Red Bank, New Jersey, and grew up near the shores of the Atlantic, living mostly in Cambridge, Massachusetts and for some years in Maine. She moved to Walla Walla, Washington, in 1997. Gerard Manley Hopkins, Wallace Stevens, Emily Dickinson, and Ingeborg Bachmann have influenced her work; she has studied with Seamus Heaney, James Galvin, and Jorie Graham. Roberts favors Borges's sentiment that "poetry is no less serious than the other elements making up our earth." For Roberts, poetry is akin to all things fierce and sensual, yet it also invokes the spirit of the ineffable.

How Late Desire Looks, Gibbs-Smith, 1997
The Quick, University of Washington Press, 2005

STAN SANVEL RUBIN

Stan Sanvel Rubin was born in Philadelphia in 1943 and grew up in Reading. His father was a clinical psychologist for the Veteran's Administration, and his mother nurtured his early interest in poetry by reading poems to him regularly. A radio buff since childhood, Rubin's earliest reading includes John Keats, T. S. Eliot, W. B. Yeats, and most importantly Wallace Stevens; his teachers include Gerald Stern at Temple University and Robert Lowell at Harvard. Something of his interest in radio influences his writing today, given that his work situates itself in the realm of primal sound, the discipline of the line, and the way poems can live in and out of time. He lives in Port Townsend, Washington.

Midnight, State Street Press, 1985
Five Colors, Custom Words, 2004
Hidden Sequel, Barrow Street, 2006

VERN RUTSALA

Vern Rutsala was born in 1934 near McCall, Idaho, and moved to Portland shortly after the bombing of Pearl Harbor in 1941. His earliest influences were William Carlos Williams, Theodore Roethke, Elizabeth Bishop, and Weldon Kees; he studied with Kenneth O. Hanson at Reed College and Donald Justice at the University of Iowa. Rutsala's poetry is firmly dedicated to simple and essential things. He lives in Portland.

The Window, Wesleyan University Press, 1964
Laments, New Rivers Press, 1975
The Journey Begins, University of Georgia Press, 1976
Paragraphs, Wesleyan University Press, 1978
Walking Home from the Icehouse, Carnegie Mellon University Press, 1981
Backtracking, Story Line Press, 1985
Ruined Cities, Carnegie Mellon University Press, 1987
Selected Poems, Story Line Press, 1991
Little-Known Sports, University of Massachusetts Press, 1994
A Handbook for Writers, White Pine Press, 2004
The Moment's Equation, Ashland Poetry Press, 2004
How We Spent Our Time, University of Akron Press, 2006

JAY RUZESKY

Born in 1965 in Edmonton, Alberta, Jay Ruzesky moved to Victoria to attend university. There he studied with John Lent and began reading the poets who would influence his work most: Sharon Olds, Don McKay, P. K. Page, and Elizabeth Bishop. His poetry is characterized by a disarming directness and a desire to praise the fact of being alive.

Am I Glad to See You, Thistledown Press, 1992
Painting the Yellow House Blue, House of Anansi Press, 1994
Blue Himalayan Poppies, Nightwood, 2001

RALPH SALISBURY

Born in 1926 of mixed blood—Cherokee, Shawnee, and English—Ralph Salisbury grew up under the influence of a banjo-playing father who introduced him to ballad literature and an Irish mother who told stories of hard times, persecution, and grief. He attended a one-room rural school in Oregon and after World War II studied with Robert Lowell, R. V. Cassill, and Paul Engle. At the center of his writing is an urgency to keep his heritage alive and accessible.

Rainbows of Stone, University of Arizona Press, 2000
War in the Genes, Cherry Grove, 2006

MAXINE SCATES

A fifth-generation Angeleno, Maxine Scates was born in Los Angeles in 1949, and moved to Eugene, Oregon, in 1973 to attend graduate school. She was influenced earliest by Ann Stanford, whose selected poems she has co-edited, as well as by Adrienne Rich, W. S. Merwin, and Denise Levertov. Drawn to poetry because the associative form of the poem lends a coherence and shapeliness to her past and present, Scates sees poetry as a way of portraying a direct response to that living.

Toluca Street, University of Pittsburgh Press, 1989
Black Loam, Cherry Grove Collections, 2005

PETER SEARS

Peter Sears was born in New York City in 1937 and moved to Oregon in 1974 to teach at Reed College. He read T. S. Eliot and Wallace Stevens early on in his writing life and as of late has been influenced by work of Pablo Neruda. In the early seventies he attended the University of Iowa Writer's Workshop and studied with Richard Hugo, Donald Justice, and Marvin Bell. His poetry is interested in intensity and is composed in a style that is direct and earnest. He lives in Corvallis, Oregon.

Tour, Breitenbush Books, 1986
The Brink, Gibbs Smith, 1999

TOM SEXTON

Born in 1940 in Lowell, Massachusetts, Tom Sexton first came to Alaska in the 1950s while serving in the U.S. Army. When he left in 1960, he never expected to return; however, eight years later he drove back to Alaska with his wife of two weeks to attend the University of Alaska. They have made their home in Alaska ever since.

Autumn in the Alaska Range, Salmon Publishing, 2000
The Lowell Poems, Adastra Press, 2005

PEGGY SHUMAKER

Peggy Shumaker was born in 1952 in La Mesa, California. She grew up in Tucson, Arizona, and moved to Fairbanks, Alaska, in 1985 to teach at the University of Alaska. Interested in collaboration, she has worked with the painter Kesler Woodward, combining his birch portraits with her poems. Her work is reflective of her desert upbringing and interior Alaska life and celebrates the need for open spaces in all our lives.

Esperanza's Hair, University of Alabama Poetry Series, 1985
The Circle of Totems, University of Pittsburgh Press, 1988
Wings Moist from the Other World, University of Pittsburgh Press, 1994
Underground Rivers, Red Hen Press, 2002
Blaze, Red Hen Press, 2005

MARTHA SILANO

Martha Silano was born and raised in Metuchen, New Jersey, where she attended public schools and, thanks to the Roberts English Series, was exposed to the poetry of Robert Frost, Edgar Allan Poe, and Emily Dickinson, among others. She received her BA from Grinnell College in 1983. After much hiking, travel, course work in biology, and working office jobs, she entered the University of Washington in 1991. She studied primarily with David Wagoner and Heather McHugh. Silano wants her poems to be an antidote to the everyday, work-a-day life.

What the Truth Tastes Like, Nightshade Press, 1999
Blue Positive, Steel Toe Books, 2006

FLOYD SKLOOT

Floyd Skloot was born in Brooklyn in 1947, the son of a kosher chicken butcher and a former radio singer. He began writing poetry in 1968 and went on to study for two years with the Irish poet Thomas Kinsella. Skloot considers his strongest poetic influences to be Robert Frost, Robert Lowell, T. S. Eliot, Elizabeth Bishop, Theodore Roethke, Dylan Thomas, and the generation of Irish poets whose voices emerged in the fifties and sixties: Kinsella, John Montague, Richard Murphy, Seamus Heaney. Skloot moved to Oregon in 1984 and was disabled in 1988 by a virus that targeted his brain. After fourteen years living near Amity, Oregon, he now lives in Portland. He calls poetry his "cornerstone."

Music Appreciation, University of Florida Press, 1994
The Evening Light, Story Line Press, 2001
The Fiddler's Trance, Bucknell University Press, 2001
Approximately Paradise, Tupelo Press, 2005
The End of Dreams, Louisiana State University Press, 2006

ESTA SPALDING

Born in Boston, raised in Hawaii, Esta Spaulding moved to Canada with her mother and sister when she was a teenager, and has lived in Vancouver since 1987. Dropping out of academia, she took a job teaching inner-city high school students and began to write poetry. Her influences at the time included W. B. Yeats, Sylvia Plath, Sharon Olds, and Adam Zagajewski. A screenwriter, she has written for CBC television. Spaulding's poems are vigorous and cinematic and have the swirl of Renaissance miniatures.

Carrying Place, House of Anansi Press, 1995
Anchoress, House of Anansi Press / Bloodaxe, 1997
Lost August, House of Anansi Press, 1999
The Wife's Account, House of Anansi Press, 2002

PRIMUS ST. JOHN

Born in Harlem in 1939 and raised in the Corona community of New York City, Primus St. John was one of the first members of his West Indian family to be born in the United States. He first came to the West as a boy scout attending a national jamboree and returned in the sixties to study briefly with William Stafford and later to attend Lewis & Clark College, where he studied with Vern Rutsala. In addition to Stafford, his earliest influences include Robert Frost, Jean Toomer, Lucille Clifton, and Maxine Kumin. For St. John, poetry is a form of play, a playground, he says, "like the one on 34th Avenue and Junction Boulevard, where I swung high, teeter-tottered with what I loved and risked my allowance on my outside shot or my drive to the basket."

Skins on the Earth, Copper Canyon Press, 1976
Love Is Not a Consolation; It Is a Light,
   Carnegie Mellon University Press, 1982
Dreamer, Carnegie Mellon University Press, 1990
Communion, Copper Canyon Press, 1999

CLEMENS STARCK

Born in 1937 in Rochester, New York, Clemens Starck first came to the Northwest during the fifties on a freight train, working jobs with the railroad, and later worked cattle ranches in Eastern Oregon. He eventually settled in the Willamette Valley and has made his living as a carpenter. He was influenced by the Modern poets early on—T. S. Eliot, Ezra Pound, and William Carlos Williams, especially—and later discovered classical Chinese poetry in translation. Starck has said that, for him, poetry is "a trick of making something as insubstantial as a piece of language appear solid and durable."

Journeyman's Wages, Story Line Press, 1995
Studying Russian on Company Time, Silverfish Review Press, 1999
China Basin, Story Line Press, 2002

LISA M. STEINMAN

Lisa M. Steinman was born in 1950, in Connecticut. Her parents worked and taught at the University of Connecticut. After attending Cornell, Steinman moved to Portland in 1976 to teach at Reed College. She read *The Golden Treasury of Verse* as a young girl and later studied with William Matthews and A. R. Ammons. Steinman's poetry is an examination of clarity in living and in language.

Lost Poems, Ithaca House, 1976
All That Comes To Light, Arrowood Books, 1989
A Book of Other Days, Arrowood Books, 1993
Carslaw's Sequences, University of Tampa Press, 2003

SANDRA STONE

Sandra Stone's childhood summers were spent in Los Angeles and at the Oregon coast; her early school years in Seattle, in view of Puget Sound. Bougainvillea, rain, dark waters, and the lingo of two opposing cities influence her poems. Today, she collaborates with architects on concepts and literary texts to create a poetic voice in public spaces.

Cocktails with Breughel at the Museum Café,
   Cleveland State University Press, 1997

JOAN SWIFT

Born in Rochester, New York, in 1926, Joan Swift grew up there and in a small coal-mining town in northern Pennsylvania's Allegheny Mountains. She began writing poems at the age of five in Rochester and continued through high school, where one of her major influences was Edna St. Vincent Millay. Later she studied alongside William Styron and Guy Davenport at Duke University. In 1957, marriage brought her to the Seattle area, where she has lived ever since, studying with Theodore Roethke in the last class he taught at the University of Washington. Swift sees poetry as a means to understand the world, even remaking it. She lives in Edmonds, Washington.

This Element, Swallow, 1965

Parts of Speech, Confluence Press, 1978
The Dark Path of Our Names, Dragon Gate, 1985
The Tiger Iris, BOA Editions, 1999

MARY SZYBIST

Mary Szybist was born near the Susquehanna River in Williamsport, Pennsylvania, in 1970. She was first drawn to poetry by the work of Theodore Roethke and later lived and studied in Iowa City, Iowa, where she taught public high school. Her poetry is a yearning for endless possibilities in language and a method of paying attention. She moved to Portland in 2004 to teach at Lewis & Clark College.

Granted, Alice James Books, 2003

SHARON THESEN

Born in Tisdale, Saskatchewan, Sharon Thesen moved to British Columbia in 1952. By the sixties she was living in Vancouver, where she worked for a few years at a radio station before attending Simon Fraser University. Robin Blaser, who had recently arrived in Canada from San Francisco, was one of her most influential teachers. Poetry, for Thesen, is the most accurate expression of human sanity. She lives in the British Columbia interior.

Artemis Hates Romance, Coach House Press, 1980
Holding the Pose, Coach House Press, 1983
Confabulations: Poems for Malcolm Lowry, Oolichan Books, 1984
The Beginning of the Long Dash, Coach House Press, 1987
The Pangs of Sunday, McClelland and Stewart, 1990
Aurora, Coach House Press, 1995
News & Smoke: Selected Poems, Talon Books, 1999
A Pair of Scissors, House of Anansi Press, 2000
The Good Bacteria, House of Anansi Press, 2006

NANCE VAN WINCKEL

Born in Roanoke, Virginia, in 1951, Nance Van Winckel moved fourteen times before finishing high school in Wisconsin. Her childhood swirled with poetry—writing rhyming ditties and song ballads or hiding poems in tree stumps. She read widely among the Beat poets, then Walt Whitman, followed by James Dickey, Sylvia Plath, Wallace Stevens, and of late European poets such as Thomas Transtromer, Georg Trakl, and Jean Follain. Van Winckel's family moved to Spokane in 1970 and has lived there ever since. She and her husband have lived there since 1990. Her poems are a bridge into and out of the lived world.

Bad Girl, with Hawk, University of Illinois Press, 1987
The Dirt, Miami University Press, 1994
After a Spell, Miami University Press, 1998
Beside Ourselves, Miami University Press, 2003

KAREN VOLKMAN

Karen Volkman was born in 1967 in Miami, Florida. She was seduced early on by poets of dense and intricate sound structures—John Keats, Dylan Thomas, Gerard Manley Hopkins, the early books of Robert Lowell, and Richard Hugo. She has said that coming to write poetry was akin to a "revelation which struck me with an actual physical shock . . . a part of my mind I never knew existed, and might never have known if I hadn't started writing." Volkman has lived in Missoula since 2004.

Crash's Law, W.W. Norton, 1996
Spar, University of Iowa Press, 2002

DAVID WAGONER

David Wagoner was born in Massillon, Ohio, in 1926, and grew up in Whiting, Indiana. He attended Penn State University, where he studied with Theodore Roethke, and later joined Roethke as a faculty member at the University of Washington. Wagoner was editor of *Poetry Northwest* for over three decades. He has said that his single most life-changing experience was moving from one of the most densely polluted areas in the U.S.—between Gary, Indiana, and Chicago—to the as yet relatively unpolluted region between the Cascade Mountains and the Pacific Ocean. A prolific poet and novelist, Wagoner's poems explore the intersection between intimacy and alienation.

Dry Sun, Dry Wind, Indiana University Press, 1953
A Place to Stand, Indiana University Press, 1958
The Nesting Ground, Indiana University Press, 1963
Staying Alive, Indiana University Press, 1966
New and Selected Poems, Indiana University Press, 1969
Riverbed, Indiana University Press, 1974
Collected Poems, Indiana University Press, 1976
Who Shall Be the Sun? Indiana University Press, 1978
In Broken Country, Atlantic-Little, Brown, 1981
First Light, Atlantic-Little, Brown, 1983
Through the Forest: New and Selected Poems, 1977–1987,
  Atlantic Monthly Press, 1987
Walt Whitman Bathing, University of Illinois Press, 1996

Traveling Light: Collected and New Poems,
  University of Illinois Press, 1999
The House of Song, University of Illinois Press, 2002
Good Morning and Good Night, University of Illinois Press, 2005

EMILY WARN

Emily Warn was born in San Francisco in 1953, and moved at the age of seven from a then-Bohemian neighborhood in Marin to an Orthodox Jewish community in Detroit. In high school, she discovered T. S. Eliot and Theodore Roethke at a time when she was rebelling against Jewish orthodoxy. For Warn, poetry snarls music and meaning every bit as powerfully and as oddly as religious traditions do, inventing complicated, invisible relations. She moved to the Pacific Northwest in 1978 to work for North Cascades National Park, and a year later moved to Seattle where she has lived, more or less, ever since.

The Leaf Path, Copper Canyon Press, 1982
The Novice Insomniac, Copper Canyon Press, 1996

INGRID WENDT

Born in Aurora, Illinois, in 1944, Ingrid Wendt moved to Eugene, Oregon, in 1966 to attend graduate school and has lived there, mostly, ever since. Weaned on Mother Goose and Robert Louis Stevenson's *A Child's Garden of Verses,* influenced early by Dylan Thomas and Theodore Roethke, trained as a classical pianist from the age of six, Wendt turned to poetry at Cornell College in Iowa, where she studied with Robert Dana, and later, at the University of Oregon, with Ralph Salisbury. Wendt's poems seek out the intersection of the passionate and the sublime. She lives in Eugene.

Moving the House, BOA Editions, 1980
Singing the Mozart Requiem, Breitenbush, 1987
The Angle of Sharpest Ascending, Word Press, 2004
Surgeonfish, WordTech Editions, 2005

JOHN WITTE

John Witte was born in upstate New York and grew up in the New Jersey suburbs. He was drawn to the Northwest by its beauty and openness, finding it less emotionally and aesthetically constraining than the East Coast. He was influenced by Ted Hughes's *Crow,* Hans Magnus Enzensberger's *Mausoleum,* and, lately, Anne Carson's translations of the fragments of Sappho. For Witte, poetry is a correction of an imbalance, using language to fill a void within the self.

Loving the Days, Wesleyan University Press, 1979
The Hurtling, Orchises Press, 2005

CAROLYNE WRIGHT

Carolyne Wright was born in Bellingham, Washington, in 1949, and grew up in Seattle, where she now lives. Her father was a banker, her mother a secretary. Her earliest reading in poetry included the work of Galway Kinnell, W. S. Merwin, Donald Justice, William Stafford, and James Wright; she later read Carolyn Kizer and Maxine Kumin. She studied with Elizabeth Bishop and, most importantly, Madeline DeFrees. Traveling in Chile in the early seventies has been a cornerstone of her self-conception as a poet, and she has translated Chilean poets, as well as a great many Bengali woman poets and writers.

Premonitions of an Uneasy Guest, Hardin-Simmons University Press,
   1983
Stealing the Children, Ahsahta Press, 1992
Seasons of Mangoes and Brainfire,
   Eastern Washington University Press, 2000
A Change of Maps, Lost Horse Press, 2006

ROBERT WRIGLEY

Robert Wrigley was born in 1951 in East St. Louis, Illinois, and grew up in coal-mining country. Following a discharge from the Army in 1971 as a conscientious objector, he came to the Northwest to attend graduate school at the University of Montana, where he studied with Richard Hugo and Madeline DeFrees. Influenced by Robert Frost, Edwin Muir, James Wright, W. S. Merwin, and John Haines, Wrigley's writing is akin to the paintings of Thomas Hart Benton—striking narratives with sweeping commonsense, a mixture of conversation and argumentation. He lives in the woods outside Moscow, Idaho.

The Sinking of Clay City, Copper Canyon Press, 1979
Moon in a Mason Jar, University of Illinois Press, 1986
What My Father Believed, University of Illinois Press, 1991
In the Bank of Beautiful Sins, Penguin, 1995
Reign of Snakes, Penguin, 1999
Lives of the Animals, Penguin, 2003
Earthly Meditations: New & Selected Poems, Penguin, 2006

DERK WYNAND

Born in 1944 in Bad Suderode, Germany, Wynand immigrated to Vancouver with his family in 1952 when his father found work as an engineer. His earliest influences include James Joyce, Franz Kafka, Samuel Beckett, Paul Celan, and Jorge Luis Borges. He took up writing poems under the tutelage of J. Michael Yates at the University of British Columbia in the late sixties. His work is noted for reevaluating the world as it is—and some of this interest comes from extensive traveling in Portugal and Mexico. Wynand lives in Victoria.

Snowscapes, The Sono Nis Press, 1974
Pointwise, Fiddlehead Poetry Books, 1980
Second Person, Sono Nis Press, 1983
Fetishistic, The Porcupine's Quill, 1984
Heat Waves, Oolichan, 1988
Closer to Home, Brick Books, 1997
Dead Man's Float, Brick Books, 2002

PATRICIA YOUNG

The daughter of Scottish and English immigrants, Patricia Young was born in Victoria, B.C., in 1954. She studied with P. K. Page and Derk Wynand, and her writing—with its direct, earthy style—has been influenced by Gwendolyn MacEwen and Margaret Atwood. Young lives in Victoria.

Travelling the Floodwaters, Turnstone Press, 1983
Melancholy Ain't No Baby, Ragweed Press, 1985
All I Ever Needed Was a Beautiful Room, Oolichan, 1987
The Mad and Beautiful Mothers, Ragweed Press, 1989
Those Were the Mermaid Days, Ragweed Press, 1991
More Watery Still, House of Anansi Press, 1993
What I Remember From My Time on Earth, House of Anansi Press, 1997
Ruin and Beauty: New and Selected Poems, House of Anansi Press, 2000

☒   ACKNOWLEDGEMENTS

Judith Barrington: "Souls Underwater" previously appeared in *He Drew Down Blue from the Sky to Make a River: The Arvon International Poetry Competition Anthology* (Arvon Foundation, 2004).

John Barton: "The Piano" previously appeared in *Vintages* 1995 (Kingston: Quarry Press, 1995); "Warhol" previously appeared in *The Fiddlehead*.

Marvin Bell: "Why Do You Stay Up So Late?" appeared on the Born website and in *Shakespeare's Wages*, Carlsen Fine Print Editions, copyright © Marvin Bell 2004. "People Walking in Fog" appeared in *Ploughshares*, copyright © Marvin Bell 2005.

James Bertolino: "Grown Men" copyright © 2002 by James Bertolino. Reprinted from *Pocket Animals*, with permission of the author and Egress Studio Press.

Linda Bierds: "Lautrec" previously appeared in *The Journal* and in *The Ghost Trio*, Henry Holt, 1994, reprinted with permission of the author; "Memento of the Hours" previously appeared in *The New Yorker* and in *The Ghost Trio*, Henry Holt, 1994, reprinted with permission of the author; "Shawl" previously appeared in *Columbia: A Magazine of Verse* and in *The Profile Makers*, Henry Holt, 1997, reprinted with permission of the author; "The Three Trees" previously appeared in *The New Yorker* and in *The Profile Makers*, Henry Holt, 1997, reprinted with permission of the author; "Van Leeuwenhoek, 1675" previously appeared in *The Threepenny Review* and in *The Profile Makers*, Henry Holt, 1997, reprinted with permission of the author.